PRAISE for *Establishing, Managing, and Protecting Your Online Reputation: A Social Media Guide for Physicians and Medical Practices*

"As the digital era inevitably invades the medical cocoon, there is a vital unmet need for physicians to adapt, especially to new challenges such as dealing with one's online reputation. Kevin Pho, a leader in the convergence of social media and healthcare, with Susan Gay, provide a comprehensive and extremely useful roadmap for doctors . . . Instead of default, sitting duck status, this information and perspective enables physicians to take charge."

ERIC TOPOL, MD

Author, *Creative Destruction of Medicine*
Scripps Clinic and The Scripps Research Institute
La Jolla, CA

"The Harrison's of social media."

DAVIS LIU, MD

Author, *Stay Healthy, Live Longer, Spend Wisely*
Sacramento, CA

"With new technology comes new challenges, and that's especially true for medical practice managers as they look to evolve their practices in innovative and responsible ways. Social media channels, physician-rating sites, and other digital communities can directly affect your practice's online reputation—and reputation management is now within the purview of the practice management profession. But where do you start and how do you go about influencing something as nebulous, fast-changing, and splintered as online reputation? This book provides practice managers with the tools they need to feel more informed and equipped to take actionable steps recommended by some of the industry's leading experts."

SUSAN L. TURNEY, MD, MS, FACMPE, FACP

MGMA President and CEO
Englewood, CO

"An insightful and thought-provoking examination of the changing landscape of medicine, filled with practical advice for clinicians."

JEROME GROOPMAN, MD, AND PAMELA HARTZBAND, MD

Authors, *Your Medical Mind: How to Choose What Is Right for You*
Brookline, MA

"I Google myself periodically, which has taught me about some of the misinformation on doctor review sites. I've since corrected a few errors. Now I realize I should do it more often and am considering starting a LinkedIn account! This book gave me a new perspective on the relationship between doctors and social media. For those of us who feel timid, the authors remind us that we already have online profiles—written by other people. The authors give us easy, practical advice to help us manage our profiles and prepare ourselves to interact with our patients in a virtual community within which we already live."

MOLLIE DAVIS, MD, MPH

Physician, Internal Medicine and Pediatrics
Johns Hopkins Community Physicians
Baltimore, MD

"For the physician contemplating the use of social media, this lovely volume is a precious and invaluable guide."

ABRAHAM VERGHESE, MD, MACP
Professor and Senior Associate Chair for the Theory and Practice of Medicine
Author, *Cutting for Stone*
Stanford University School of Medicine
Stanford, CA

"This book is sensational. It provides an argument that wins hands-down on how doctors no longer have the luxury of ignoring social media and its impact. This book will help physicians understand and prepare themselves for social media's impact on their future."

JUDY CAPKO
Founder, Capko & Company
Author, *Secrets of the Best-Run Practices*, 2nd Edition
Thousand Oaks, CA

"*Establishing, Managing, and Protecting Your Online Reputation: A Social Media Guide for Physicians and Medical Practices* is a primer on the essentials about why your medical digital footprint is important and how to best manage it. This must-read book also chronicles the path of Dr. Pho from the beginnings as an internal medicine physician and patient advocate from New Hampshire to today as social media's leading physician voice via his very popular website, KevinMD.com."

MIKE SEVILLA, MD
Family Practice Center of Salem
Salem, OH

"Medical practice reputation and branding by social media has been on my high-priority list. This book will be significant for every healthcare executive, physician leader, and governing board member! The content is clear, concise, and highly informative. It summarizes benefits, business opportunities, and threats, and provides specific go-to resources. The content calls out social media influences, both positive and negative, generating an awareness of the need to address the opportunities and risks immediately. The case examples are brief and resonate with the must-do implementation of policy and guideline structure within the practice and for physician members. This implementation planning guide responds not only to the 'business' of medicine but to the progression to regulatory-mandated transparency.

The time investment in reading (significantly quick and interesting . . . not tedious in any manner) becomes a double payback. I found it stimulated me to take immediate action while the information was fresh, and I plan to keep it close at hand as a bookshelf resource reference and coaching material as my social media policies and procedures evolve. Dr. Pho and Ms. Gay have provided the busy healthcare executive with the toolkit of content for governance regarding social media exposure and a comprehensive resource list to build the policies.

After reading this material, I was curious about and compelled to immediately investigate the resources suggested. I was astonished at what I learned about our practice at social media sites. No more resting on our "reputation and laurels" of 26+ years of community contribution and service!

I recommend that every administrator read this book, and I suggest that it be distributed to governing boards to better clarify their understanding of discussions of opportunities and threats evolving with social media to include those involving patients and staff. In summary, this is a very timely, noteworthy book and a must read to understand the critical business knowledge required to manage the impact of social media on the medical practice industry!"

REBECCA S. DEAN, MA, FACMPE

Chief Executive Officer
Sportsmedicine & Orthopaedics Fairbanks
Fairbanks, AK

"Every physician and practice marketing manager will find value in this book—from the techno-skeptic to the sophisticate. You'll get perspectives and references that will help you form your own online strategy. I know I did!"

KAREN ZUPKO

Karen Zupko & Associates
Chicago, IL

"A doctor's greatest strength is his or her reputation. We spend our entire professional lives creating and protecting this valuable asset. Dr. Pho and Ms. Gay have provided the necessary steps and techniques to guard and protect your online reputation. I highly recommend their book and believe that everyone who reads it will have the tools and techniques to keep their reputation polished and pristine."

NEIL BAUM, MD

Author, *Marketing Your Clinical Practices: Ethically, Effectively, Economically,* 4th Edition
Clinical Associate Professor of Urology
Tulane Medical School
New Orleans, LA

"Social media is here to stay! *Establishing, Managing, and Protecting Your Online Reputation* is a must-have book for every physician and/or medical practice involved in social media. Dr. Pho (KevinMD.com) has once again proven that his knowledge is valuable in today's technology-driven world. I would highly recommend every medical office manager and physician read this book before getting heavily involved in social media!"

DESIREE R. BAYLIN, CPM, CHRS, COM

Executive Director
Physician Office Managers Association of America (POMAA)
Dallastown, PA

"It takes a lifetime to build a reputation but only a single act, blog, e-mail, online comment, Facebook post, texted picture, or tweet to destroy it. That's because online communication may go massive instantly. And it's the reason the 'mainstream' media, including medical journals and medical television, have editors and peer reviewers and build in a delay factor. Keeping egg off authors' faces, protecting authors from themselves, and protecting readers are key roles for editors and peer reviewers.

Physicians want to succeed. They often adopt new technology very quickly if it will help them do their jobs better and faster, and especially if it generates new revenue. If not, they wisely drag their feet. They became rapid adapters of Internet 1.0, one-way communication, rapid digital access to the world literature. But physicians have been very slow at adopting Internet 2.0, bi- and multi-directional messaging. They like to speak; to listen, not so much. To judge, a great deal; to be judged, very little.

However, social media will not go away. In some form, or many forms, it is here to stay. And it refuses to be ignored. Most of the social spheres have adopted it; many have embraced it. It can bite you, doctor, badly, and you may not even know it unless you are plugged in. It may be as virulent to your reputation and welfare as rabies, and there is no vaccine, save your informed involvement.

This book is the newest, most comprehensive, most detailed and up-to-date reference source available to American physicians and medical practices. Richly nuanced by America's most popular and authoritative physician blogger and social media expert, it can guide you through this swamp—maybe not clean, but ready to move forward."

GEORGE D. LUNDBERG, MD

Editor in Chief, CollabRx
Editor at Large, MedPage Today
President, The Lundberg Institute
Consulting Professor, Stanford University
Los Gatos, CA

"*Establishing, Managing, and Protecting Your Online Reputation: A Social Media Guide for Physicians and Medical Practices* is written as both an educational and instructional tool to help medical practitioners understand and manage their online reputation in the medical sector. In today's world, this is absolutely crucial, and these authors have simplified the process. This is a must-read for medical practitioners and all others in the medical field."

CHAD SCHWARZ

President/CEO
Integrated MedReps, LLC
Morganville, NJ

"Social media is the wave of the future in medicine, and I can't think of a doctor more qualified to write about this phenomenon than Kevin Pho. This book is essential reading for any doctor or medical practice looking to establish an online presence."

SANDEEP JAUHAR, MD

Author, *Intern: A Doctor's Initiation*
Long Island Jewish Medical Center
Department of Cardiology
New Hyde Park, NY

"In this new online social media age, it is imperative that everyone, but most especially professionals looking to build, grow, and maintain a business or a practice, establish a good reputation online. And even more importantly, to make sure that their online presence is properly monitored and maintained, as this can be the life blood of their business and can truly provide a 'make it or break it' opportunity. I would recommend that all physicians, no matter where they are in building their practice, or even for those who already have a well-established practice, read this book and strongly consider the excellent ideas and direction it could take their practice."

REED TINSLEY, CPA, CVA, CFP, CHBC

A Houston-Based CPA and Certified Healthcare Business Consultant
Houston, TX

"As one of the most prolific practitioners in the world of social media, Kevin Pho's insights for doctors and other health professionals are soundly based on experience. His ability to demystify this arena for others comes from a clear and concise exposition of what is fact and what is fear. His book is an important contribution to creating a more patient-centric healthcare system that is also highly respectful of the knowledge and good intentions of physicians and other clinicians."

PAUL F. LEVY

Former CEO, Beth Israel Deaconess Medical Center
Author, *Goal Play! Leadership Lessons from the Soccer Field*
Newton, MA

"Dr. Kevin Pho is a modern legend of healthcare-related social media. His website, KevinMD.com, is the go-to physician blog for healthcare information. Dr. Pho has compiled his years of experience and knowledge into a fantastic book that should be considered required reading for all doctors. Social media is the future of doctor–patient communication, and this book provides a comprehensive guide to navigating the social media arena. From LinkedIn to Facebook, to Twitter, to Google+, readers will learn how to become the maestro of their online reputation, marketing, and communication with patients. Very highly recommended!"

ANTHONY YOUN, MD, FACS

YOUN Plastic Surgery, PLLC
Troy, MI

"This book provides valuable insight to physicians and their staff . . . a virtual roadmap to navigate the digital age of establishing a positive online presence, developing marketing strategies, and addressing social media identities. It's a must-read for today's 21st century digital medical practice!"

REBECCA UMBERGER, CMA (AAMA), CPM

Aultman MSO, Aultman Hospital
Maternal and Fetal Management
Canton, OH

"The insights that Dr. Pho and Ms. Gay share in their book are instrumental in learning how social media will impact an outpatient practice and more importantly the physician's reputation. They provide great content and examples to help physicians have a strong and positive Internet presence. A must-read for healthcare administrators and healthcare providers."

DANIELLE DEMAIO-DEANGELIS, MHA, COPM

Administrator
Jefferson University Physicians
Department of Otolaryngology-Head and Neck Surgery
Philadelphia, PA

"For private practice physicians, reputation management is here to stay. In this ground-breaking book, Kevin Pho and Susan Gay provide you with the language, the players, and the smart techniques to take control of your reputation online. The energy of these authors (and their purpose) translates into winning techniques you can use in your own practice. The book includes practical stories and up-to-date references. It is beautifully researched and edited. Take control of your own reputation now!"

JOHN GUILIANA, DPM, MS, AND HAL ORNSTEIN, DPM, FASPS

Authors, *31½ Essentials for Running Your Medical Practice*
Blairstown, NJ, and Howell, NJ

"*Establishing, Managing, and Protecting Your Online Reputation: A Social Media Guide for Physicians and Medical Practices* could not have come at a better time. Dr. Kevin Pho and Susan Gay have written a book that will be a great service for practice administrators and business managers. Administrators know physician reputation has an impact on the success of the practice. We also know that monitoring and managing the physician reputation is a growing concern for all medical practices. Patients don't look for doctors in the Yellow Pages like they used to! Now it is all online. Read this book and you'll have the both the inspiration and a blueprint to help your doctors with this new element of medical practice. The case studies of how other physicians manage their reputation are particularly useful, as are the extra resources in the Appendix."

TODD BLUM, MHA, MBA, CMPE
Chief Executive Officer
Ear, Nose and Throat Associates of South Florida
Boca Raton, FL

"Social media is a powerful tool to help you build relationships with new patients and deepen relationships with people who know you. This book shows you 'online bedside manners' that will get you off on the right foot."

VICKI RACKNER, MD
President, www.medicalbridges.com
Seattle, WA

"We live in a very interesting time—a period of rapidly accelerating change and transformation in how human beings communicate in fundamentally different and infinitely more powerful new ways. Dr. Pho and Ms. Gay demonstrate a deep understanding of how this phenomenon is affecting medical practitioners and offer a clear-eyed approach with specific strategies to empower doctors to use these new media to build and support their personal brands in their markets. In an age when most doctors are not even aware of the critical need to manage their reputation online, and some are even being extorted with threats of reputation attacks, *Establishing, Managing, and Protecting Your Online Reputation: A Social Media Guide for Physicians and Medical Practices* offers the most comprehensive and positive approach to managing and protecting our precious online reputations that I have seen. Managing your online reputation is not something physicians can opt out of. This new work is their guide to ensuring they protect their good name now and in the future."

REM JACKSON
President and CEO
Top Practices
Lititz, PA

"Social media and online information are embedded in our culture and getting more so every day. Informed consumers, including payers and patients, use the Internet to research potential providers. This book will take you from an understanding of the basics to developing usage strategies. It will also help you recognize the negative aspects, including damage to provider reputations and what can be done to prevent and repair this when it occurs."

STEVEN NELSON, CPA
Chief Financial Officer
Panorama Orthopedics & Spine Center
Golden, CO

"Dr. Pho's book provides great insight into online reputations. For those who are uncertain about an online presence, he suggests methods to become more familiar with social media, such as lurking. The book is very well laid out and covers almost anything you could want to know about social media and your online reputation. It's a good read for those who are new to social media as well as to those who want to take it to the next level!"

MELISSA J. PITCHFORD, CPA
Chief Financial Officer
Katzen Eye Group
Baltimore, MD

ESTABLISHING, MANAGING, *and* PROTECTING YOUR ONLINE REPUTATION

A Social Media Guide for Physicians and Medical Practices

By Kevin Pho, MD, and Susan Gay

FOREWORD BY ROBERT M. WACHTER, MD

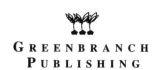

GREENBRANCH
PUBLISHING

PO Box 208
Phoenix, MD 21131
Phone: (800) 933-3711
Fax: (410) 329-1510
Email: info@greenbranch.com
Website: www.greenbranch.com, www.mpmnetwork.com, www.soundpractice.net, www.codapedia.com

No patent liability is assumed with respect to the use of the information contained herein. Although every precaution has been taken in the preparation of this book, the publisher and the authors assume no responsibility for errors or omissions. Nor is any liability assumed from damages resulting from the use of the information contained herein. For information, Greenbranch Publishing, PO Box 208, Phoenix, MD 21131.

All terms mentioned in this book that are known to be or are suspected of being trademarks or service marks have been appropriately capitalized. Greenbranch Publishing cannot attest to the accuracy of this information. Use of a term in this book should not be regarded as affecting the validity of the trademark or service mark. The fact that an organization or website is referred to in this work as a citation and/or a potential source of further information does not mean that the author or publisher endorses the information the organization or website may provide or recommendations it may make. Further, readers should be aware that internet websites listed in this work may have changed or disappeared between when this work was written and when it is read.

The strategies contained herein may not be suitable for every situation. This publication is designed to provide general medical practice management information and is sold with the understanding that neither the author nor the publisher is engaged in rendering legal, accounting, ethical, or clinical advice. If legal or other expert advice is required, the services of a competent professional person should be sought.

Greenbranch Publishing books are available at special quantity discounts for bulk purchases as premiums, fund-raising, or educational use. info@greenbranch.com or (800) 933-3711.

13   8 7 6 5 4 3 2 1

Interpretation of the printing code: The rightmost number of the first series of numbers is the year of the book's printing; the rightmost number of the second series of numbers is the number of printing. For example, a printing code of 13-1 shows that the first printing occurred in 2013.

Printed in the United States of America by United Book Press, Inc.
www.unitedbookpress.com

PUBLISHER
Nancy Collins

EDITORIAL ASSISTANT
Jennifer Weiss

BOOK DESIGNER
Laura Carter
Carter Publishing Studio

INDEX
Robert A. Saigh

COPYEDITOR
Karen Doyle

PUBLISHER'S NOTE: This book offers a unique perspective on online reputation management. One of the authors (SG) had noticed the trend toward online physician reviews, and the increasing frustrations many physicians had about them, and set out to develop a practical resource to guide them. The publisher sought a leading physician author active in social media (KP), and a partnership was born. Throughout the book, Dr. Pho's personal experiences are told in the first person, amplified by contributions of other physicians, patients, and industry leaders.

Table of Contents

DEDICATION

To Mom and Dad, for the drive to pursue medicine,
and the imagination to think beyond it.

To my family, Anita, Sydney, and Kyla,
for keeping my social media journey alive
with your love, patience, and support.

K.P.

To my wonderful family—my husband, Jon, and children,
Katie and Paul Andrews—for their love and encouragement in everything I do.

To Brit B. Gay Jr., MD, who inspired my interest in medicine,
and the memory of Evelyn W. Gay, who inspired my interest in writing and
publishing, for providing me with the groundwork for a great career.

To the memory of Morgan, the Maine Coon who purred
lovingly by my side on many late nights.

S.G.

About the Authors

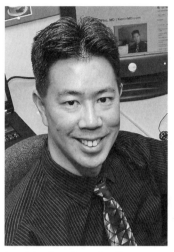

KEVIN PHO is a board-certified internal medicine physician and founder of KevinMD.com, which *Forbes* called a "must-read health blog." Klout named him the Web's top social media influencer in healthcare and medicine, and CNN named @KevinMD one of its five recommended Twitter health feeds.

Transforming his social media presence into a mainstream media voice, he has been interviewed on the "CBS Evening News with Katie Couric," and his commentary regularly appears in *USA Today*, where he is a member of its editorial Board of Contributors, as well as CNN and the *New York Times*. His opinion pieces highlight the challenges real-world doctors face, ranging from the primary care shortage to the epidemic of physician burnout.

His dual perspectives as a practicing physician and a healthcare social media leader contribute to his unique social media journey. He shares his story in keynotes nationwide, with audiences that include the PRSA Health Academy, Healthcare Internet Conference, Massachusetts Medical Society, American Academy of Otolaryngology, Texas Medical Association, National Council for Community Behavioral Healthcare, and PAINWeek.

Kevin practices primary care at Nashua Medical Group in Nashua, New Hampshire. He received his medical degree from and completed his residency at Boston University School of Medicine, and is a member of the *New Hampshire Union Leader*'s 2010 class of New Hampshire's 40 Under Forty. He lives in Nashua with his wife and two daughters. He can be contacted at KevinMD.com.

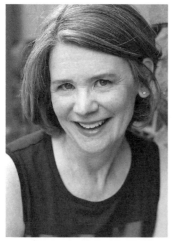 **SUSAN GAY** is a medical publisher and content strategist with over 25 years of experience in medical publishing leadership. Known for her foresight and vision in creating groundbreaking publications, she has published several hundred books, journals, and multimedia products, many of them market leaders. Her creative imprint can be seen in such pioneering works as *The 5-Minute Clinical Consult* and the Netter Collection reference works. As Vice President and Publisher at Williams & Wilkins (now Wolters Kluwer Health), Susan was the first clinical publisher to apply branding strategies to a clinical publishing program. Earlier in her career, she was an award-winning editor at Mosby and served as president of the American Medical Publishers Association.

As the digital era began to fundamentally reinvent medicine and healthcare delivery, Susan created her own firm to focus on providing multichannel content, creating greater brand awareness for professional information products, and helping publishers and societies extend their existing portfolios. She has worked with many companies and societies in the medical field including: American Medical Association, American Academy of Pediatrics, Sage Publications, Medcases, Springer, MediMedia, Lippincott Williams & Wilkins, Elsevier, Harcourt Health Sciences, and Thomson-PDR.

Through it all, Susan has had a keen eye for the forces that shape medical practice. With a knack for identifying trends, Susan is known for recruiting and collaborating with cutting-edge authors to deliver much-needed information to practicing physicians. Today, she is focused on the digital future of healthcare and all that it means for clinical medicine, medical education, and information delivery. She has leveraged her experience in creating brands of information to help individual medical practices establish their own brands on the Web. Her partnership with Kevin Pho on this book has been instrumental in shaping one of the most important emerging concepts in the practice of medicine—that of creating a personal brand through social media. She can be contacted at susan.infobrand@comcast.net.

Acknowledgments

The value of this book has been strengthened by the addition of personal stories from people who have used social media to make a positive difference in healthcare. We thank all of those who contributed their stories for taking time out of their busy lives and practices to be a part of this collaborative endeavor. Providing detailed information on the major rating sites is one of the goals of the book, and for that, we thank all those who responded to our questions. We are also grateful to Bob Wachter who not only took the time to compose a foreword, but did so in an entertaining and insightful way that perfectly places our work in the context of today's healthcare environment.

Without the unflagging support of our publisher, Nancy Collins at Greenbranch Publishing, this book would not have been possible. The text has been greatly enhanced by the striking design created by Laura Carter, the meticulous editing by Karen Doyle, and the proofreading by Jennifer Weiss. We thank Nancy and her team for giving us the opportunity to write this book and for providing encouragement, feedback, and professionalism in creating a high-quality product.

Because there are two of us, we each have people who have helped us with this project or influenced our careers.

WHEN I COMPLETED MEDICAL TRAINING A DECADE AGO, little did I know that my journey would take me to where I am now. I am deeply indebted to the many who have guided me along the way. Thank you to my friends and colleagues at Nashua Medical Group, who took a chance on a newly minted doctor and had the patience to nurture me into the physician I am today. Thanks also to Glen Nishimura, Susan Ellingwood, and Flora Zhang, who gave an unknown voice the opportunity to be heard from a national media stage. And finally, KevinMD would not exist without MedPage Today and Everyday Health, whose continuing support has been instrumental in realizing my social media vision. **K.P.**

THE SUBJECT OF ONLINE REVIEW SITES FOR PHYSICIANS has received increasing coverage in both the medical literature and popular press. One article in particular addressing doctors' frustrations with online ratings, published in the *Philadelphia Inquirer* in January 2012, sparked the idea for this book. Thanks to Stacey Burling for her balanced coverage that helped me see the need for a guide to help healthcare professionals. I would also like to express my gratitude to the many people in the medical publishing industry who, over the years, have supported my ideas and given me opportunities to pursue new and original concepts. I am especially indebted to Ted Hutton, John Gardner, Tom Mackey, and the late Sheila Carey. Finally, thanks to Paul Andrews, who provided valuable technical and editorial assistance on the social media sites included in the book. **S.G.**

Contributors

Vineet Arora, MD, MAPP
Assistant Dean, Scholarship & Discovery
University of Chicago Pritzker School of Medicine
Chicago, Illinois

Neil Baum, MD
Associate Clinical Professor
Department of Urology
Tulane Medical School
New Orleans, Louisiana

Natasha Burgert, MD
Pediatric Associates
Kansas City, Missouri

Kevin R. Campbell, MD
Wake Heart & Vascular
Raleigh, North Carolina

Jamie Cesaretti, MD, MS
Winter Park Cancer Center
Winter Park, Florida

Katherine Chretien, MD
Associate Professor
Department of Medicine
George Washington University
Washington, DC

Dave deBronkart
Blogger, Speaker, Policy Advisor
Nashua, New Hampshire

Susannah Fox
Associate Director
Pew Internet & American Life Project
Washington, DC

Nicholas Genes, MD, PhD
Assistant Professor
Department of Emergency Medicine
Mount Sinai School of Medicine
New York, New York

Bobby Ghaheri, MD
The Oregon Clinic
Portland, Oregon

Jordan Grumet, MD
Park Avenue Associates
Evanston, Illinois

Joseph Kim, MD, MPH
President
MCM Education
Newtown, Pennsylvania

Edmund Kwok, MD, FRCPC, MHA, MSc
Director of Operational & Performance
    Evaluation
Department of Emergency Medicine
University of Ottawa
Ottawa, Ontario, Canada

Davis Liu, MD
The Permanente Medical Group
Sacramento, California

Jeff Livingston, MD
MacArthur OB/GYN
Irving, Texas

Howard J. Luks, MD
University Orthopaedics
Hawthorne, New York

John M. Mandrola, MD, FACC
Baptist Medical Associates
Louisville, Kentucky

"Dr. Fizzy McFizz"
http://doccartoon.blogspot.com

Michael B. Moore
Medical Student
Pacific Northwest University of Health Sciences
Yakima, Washington

Sherry Pagoto, PhD
Associate Professor
Department of Medicine
University of Massachusetts Medical School
Worcester, Massachusetts

John Schumann, MD
Associate Professor
Department of Medicine
University of Oklahoma School of
    Community Medicine
Tulsa, Oklahoma

Christian T. Sinclair, MD, FAAHPM
National Hospice Medical Director
Overland Park, Kansas

Kerri Morrone Sparling
Writer and Patient Advocate
Coventry, Rhode Island

Wendy Sue Swanson, MD, MBE
Pediatrician, Author
Seattle Children's Hospital, The Everett Clinic
Seattle, Washington

Bryan Vartabedian, MD
Assistant Professor
Department of Pediatrics
Baylor College of Medicine
Houston, Texas

Michael A. Woo-Ming, MD, MPH
RepMD
Escondido, California

Maria Yang, MD
Medical Director, Crisis Solutions Center
DESC – Downtown Emergency Service Center
Seattle, Washington

Shara Yurkiewicz
Medical Student
Harvard Medical School
Brookline, Massachusetts

Foreword

Information technology is transforming the way we teach, learn, communicate, work, play, and think. And there are few areas in which the changes have been more deeply felt than in healthcare.

A few years ago, one prominent physician-leader told me he wouldn't read blogs. "I already have too much on my plate," he said. He reads them today. I've heard from others who once refused to use e-mail, or text messaging, or electronic health records, or Facebook, or Twitter. In every case, resistance gave way to acceptance—a digital version of Elisabeth Kübler-Ross's famous hierarchy—as the benefits became too hard to ignore. Luddite Island has become an increasingly lonely place.

While I have always been something of a technophile, I was nowhere near the leading edge of these developments. I began blogging in 2007, after realizing that I had observations I wanted to make about a variety of issues in patient safety, healthcare quality, and policy, and that my only vehicle for publishing them (or so I believed) was a traditional medical journal. It was nice when one of my articles showed up in *JAMA* or the *New England Journal of Medicine*, but the peer-review process meant a six-month lag between idea and publication (for the papers that weren't rejected!), during which most topics had grown stale.

Blogging changed all that: it shortened the path from idea to publication to a couple of days (plus none of that rejection stuff). I started tweeting in 2011, partly as a way to promote my blog, but instantly found that it greatly extended my "brand," and that there was no more fun and useful way to wait for an elevator. Today, I find that more people know me from my blog writings than from my 200 peer-reviewed articles and six books, and that I receive more direct feedback about my blog posts than about virtually any of my writings in more traditional media. Like Willie Sutton's famous line about why he robbed banks ("Because that's where the money is"), I blog and tweet because, quite simply, that is where interesting and interested people increasingly live.

The transformation of healthcare in the information age has broad consequences. Knowledge has been democratized: patients now commonly search for information from Dr. Google before they consult Dr. Welby. The idea of patients seeking support and insight from communities of individuals with similar problems—pioneered more than 75 years ago by Alcoholics Anonymous—has been adopted by groups ranging from patients with cancer to families of patients with Alzheimer's. But in today's incarnations, the meetings are online, not in the local church basement.

Not only does today's patient expect to have a virtual relationship with his or her doctor, but the data that inform this relationship—everything from the heart failure patient's daily weight to the diabetic patient's blood glucose levels—can now be wirelessly transmitted from a digital device to the physician's computer, where it can be analyzed and acted upon. In the old days, the office visit (or the hospitalization) was the fleeting interlude during which the business of doctoring was conducted. Today, these face-to-face meetings are punctuation marks in a narrative arc that is no longer bound by physical proximity.

Even with all these changes in the nature of the doctor-patient relationship, there may be none as transformative, and unsettling to physicians, as the fact that patients are increasingly learning about their doctors based on the doctors' online presence. This, of course, is not unique to medicine: we all have dual personalities today, our flesh-and-blood persona and our online persona. For many physicians—particularly those who are happy with who they are, or who have left electronic breadcrumbs behind from college fraternity or sorority parties—these developments may be cause for angst, even alarm.

But whether we like it or not, our online reputation is becoming the main prism through which we will be known—to colleagues, to friends, to patients, to prospective employers, really to everyone except our most intimate partners. With this realization comes the recognition that we can no longer afford to be passive observers of our online persona. Managing it needs to be an intentional act, both to avoid trouble and to ensure that it is an honest reflection of our best selves.

As we traverse this new and exotic waterway, we could not have a better river pilot than Dr. Kevin Pho, who in this book offers us his vast insights about this rapidly changing ecosystem. Pho, an internal medicine physician from Nashua, New Hampshire, stepped into the world of blogs, tweets, and Facebook early and skillfully, and has since cemented his role as "social media's leading physician voice." In fact, in the field of social media and healthcare, Pho has achieved the first-name-only cachet generally reserved for celebrities (Oprah, Madonna, Hillary). His copilot on this journey is Susan Gay, an experienced leader in healthcare publishing, both old-school and digital. Their book is written in plainspoken language, and it is exhaustively researched. The advice it offers is practical and can be applied today. I have already begun implementing some of it myself: the book prompted me to join LinkedIn and to Google myself.

Several years ago, I attended a meeting of the faculty in my department at the University of California, San Francisco. The discussion turned to all of the changes that were transforming the practice of medicine: new regulations, public reporting, payment methods, computerized prescribing, social media, you name it. One of my esteemed senior clinicians, someone who had done quite well under the old rules, stood up to address his colleagues, including me.

"You know," he said, "this could be worse."

I was flabbergasted—he was just the kind of graybeard to believe that all of these changes were ruining medicine, at least medicine as he knew it. But then he said: "I could be younger."

While I found his comment amusing, I also profoundly disagreed with it. To me, there has never been a more exciting time to be a healthcare professional. Yes, we are under increasing pressure to find ways to deliver the highest quality and safest care. We have recognized the need to engage patients and families in new ways. We simply must spend less money and waste fewer resources. And we have to do all these things using tools, including digital ones, that were probably not invented when we were in medical school.

While change is hard, one of the things I like about this book is its can-do spirit and optimism. Sure, as many a politician and a handful of doctors have learned, there are lines surrounding our online behavior that should not be crossed (particularly related to privacy and decorum), and some of these aren't fully drawn yet. Yes, social media can distract instead of enlighten, wrong information can look suspiciously like correct information in a tweet or blog, and e-charlatans can have successful runs before they are unmasked. Yet Pho and Gay emphasize the magnificent attractions that the digital world offers—to disseminate ideas, to forge new relationships with patients and colleagues, and to make a difference.

Like them, I believe that the benefits of social media far outweigh the hazards, for both physicians and patients. This book will help ensure that we take full advantage of these opportunities, while steering clear of the pitfalls.

ROBERT M. WACHTER, MD
Professor and Associate Chairman, Department of Medicine
University of California, San Francisco
Chair, American Board of Internal Medicine
Blog: www.wachtersworld.org
Twitter: @Bob_Wachter

Preface

"Stories unite people, theories divide them."

—James Billington, Librarian of Congress

Why is your online reputation important? Because that's where your patients go not only to get health information but to read more about you.

Social media has ushered in a new era. The use of social media has grown from 5% of all adults in 2005 to 62% worldwide today, and 46% in the United States. It has fundamentally transformed the way we communicate.

How many of us today would not look on TripAdvisor or some other travel site before booking a hotel? How many of us would buy a book or make a reservation at a restaurant without first looking at its reviews online?

Studies have shown that one-third of consumers are using social media for health-related issues. They are not just seeking information about their diseases or symptoms, but increasingly they are looking for information about physicians and hospitals. The Internet and social media are second nature to many people. Online communities allow patients with similar conditions to share stories, improve morale, and seek guidance from others who understand their plight.

Social media has opened the door for two-way communication between physicians and patients. Partnering with patients can have a profound effect on patient satisfaction and ultimately on outcomes. Social media tools help grow those relationships and allow you to share your knowledge. Physicians and other health professionals can and should either be a source of reputable information themselves or guide patients to reputable health websites.

How can social media help? It gives health professionals an opportunity to tell their stories. Stories put a human face on the evidence doctors rely on to teach and treat their patients. The power of the narrative has been the subject of numerous research studies and articles in recent years. Patients are already telling their personal stories, while medicine is largely reported in the form of evidence-based studies that tend to ignore the personal elements. While the facts are important, the ability to reach people with storytelling will become as important in bringing about healthcare change. That's where doctors can make a difference in their patients' lives—by adding a personal element such as their commentary on current media coverage of medical news or original patient education materials sent via YouTube or a blog.

Social media can be used by healthcare professionals to take the lead in creating compelling stories based on sound science to counter the often false claims popularized by celebrities and the media. In keeping with this concept, storytelling is the leitmotif of this book as well. Interspersed among reports of studies, guidelines, and recommendations are real-life experiences of patients, healthcare professionals, and industry leaders who are using social media to make a difference.

Furthermore, social media doesn't just allow you to reach out to patients by providing credible information; it can make them more satisfied too, thus boosting your online reputation. Patients who find you online are more apt to like and trust you from the start. They may come to you better prepared and be more receptive to your instructions as well. What could this mean to you? A better relationship with patients and a significantly higher online rating.

The scope of online reputation management is broader than you may think. It does not just focus on reviews posted by patients but on the coordinated efforts of government bodies and large organizations, the results of which will be widely available online.

Patient satisfaction figures prominently in several large-scale initiatives that have the potential to affect both the reputation and the bottom line of every medical practice. The federal government has taken some important steps in this direction through the policies of the Centers for Medicare & Medicaid Services. Pay models for physicians will change, and will also likely include patient satisfaction scores, in part, as a measurement of quality.

Where Medicare goes, private insurers are sure to follow. Many insurers already collect patient reviews or license information from one of the major rating sites as a service to their members. Whether those ratings ultimately affect physician payments is not known, but it is certainly within the realm of possibility. Consumer Reports is now also more heavily involved in the healthcare field with its recent release of a report on primary care practices in Massachusetts.

The economic incentives, coupled with changing demographics and readily available online tools to disseminate information, mean that there is no going back. A more transparent healthcare system is here to stay, and the use of online physician rating sites is likely to grow as well.

This book is a clarion call for establishing a strong digital footprint, so that as social media becomes even more widely used in healthcare and as government organizations expand their spotlight on patient satisfaction, your reputation will be firmly established. This book is designed to be your guide to six leading social media platforms—LinkedIn, Facebook, YouTube, Twitter, Google+, and blogs—as well as 12 of the major physician rating sites. We also present evidence on the prevalence of social media today, and we dispel the myth that all online reviews of doctors are negative.

Entire books could be written on some of the topics addressed in this book. Patient satisfaction and search engine optimization, for instance, are broad, complex areas that increasingly impact the healthcare professional. Key elements of those topics are distilled here as they relate to online reputation management.

Once you've ventured into social media, safeguarding your reputation will be an essential element of your overall strategy. We provide tips on how to monitor your reputation, respond to reviews, and maintain standards of professionalism. Proper use of social media does not just encompass what *not to do*; it includes the imperatives of what we *must do* to maintain our professional image in this new era.

We hope that you will use this guide to create your own goals for your social media presence. Some of you may want to attract more patients but some of you already have a full practice. In either case, you can extend your reach and be part of your patients' lives outside the confines of the office visit. What could be a more efficient way to positively guide patients' health when they are not in your office? What could have a more positive impact on your online reputation?

KEVIN PHO, MD
SUSAN M. GAY
January 2013

"In the long history of humankind those who learned to collaborate and improvise most effectively have prevailed."

—Charles Darwin

CHAPTER 1

Disrupting the Healthcare Landscape

SOCIAL MEDIA IS NOT A PASSING FAD

A few years ago, physicians had to learn to deal with patients doing Internet research and coming to their appointments armed with the information they found. By September 2012, 72% of adults online in the United States were using the Internet to search for health-related information.[1] These days, the Web has produced an entirely new level of consumer involvement in healthcare, through the explosive growth of social media.

What is social media? According to Wikipedia, "social media includes web-based and mobile-based technologies which are used to turn communication into interactive dialogue among organizations, communities, and individuals."[2]

The *Merriam-Webster Dictionary* defines social media as "forms of electronic communication through which users create online communities to share information, ideas, personal messages, and other content."[3]

Tim McKenna, social media specialist at the Pennsylvania Academy of Family Physicians, puts it most succinctly. He calls social media "digital word of mouth."[4]

Social media consists of websites or mobile apps that facilitate the creation and exchange of user-generated content. Examples include: a picture on Flickr, a video on YouTube, a blog post, or a status update on Facebook or Twitter. Social media's defining characteristic is that it encourages two-way communication, or in other words, conversation.

The use of social media has grown from 5% of all adults in 2005 to 62% worldwide today, and 46% of all adults in the United States.[5] Social media has fundamentally transformed the way we communicate. Many businesses, large and small, have a presence on Facebook. Every organization has to be careful about what its employees say on Twitter.

Given the interactive nature of social media, it seems only logical that some form of review component would emerge as Web 2.0 capabilities took shape. How many of us today would not look on TripAdvisor or some other travel site before booking a hotel? How many of us would buy a book or make a reservation at a restaurant without first looking at its reviews online?

In describing the 2010 report on Online Product Research from the Pew Research Center's Internet & American Life Project, author Jim Jansen concluded that "E-commerce is now a 360-degree experience for shoppers," beginning with research that leads to a purchase, that then leads to commentary and review of that purchase.[6] Today, no business can afford to ignore social media.

But what does this have to do with healthcare, you may ask?

Everything that is current and trendsetting now will eventually become relevant in healthcare—it just takes several years to happen. Consider the beeper. I still carry one when I'm on call. If someone at the hospital or a patient wants to reach me, he or she will page me, and I'll call back. In the early 1990s, the only people who had beepers were doctors and drug dealers.[7] Now it's just the doctors; the drug dealers have moved on to smartphones!

What social media sites are the most popular? The largest by far (and so far!) is Facebook, with over a billion users.[8] That's more than the population of many countries, including the United States. Twitter averages over 340 million tweets per day, has 140 million users, and is only six years old.[9] YouTube, the popular video hosting site, has more video posted monthly than all three major TV networks have produced in 60 years.[10]

Some of the most notable data center on the age of social media users. If you think only young people use social media, think again. Studies show that people over the age of 35 have increased their use of social media more than their younger counterparts. In the over-65 age group, usage has gone up 154% in the past two years![11]

To see how pervasive social media is in our culture today, consider the following:

- The average Internet user in the United States spends 32 hours online per month, and now social networking is the most popular online activity; adults spend 22% of their online time on social media channels like Facebook and Twitter.[12]
- People are using social media more than they are communicating via e-mail (19% of their time) or using search engines (21% of their time).[12]
- Smartphone owners now spend as much time using social networking apps as they do playing games—on average, 24 minutes per day.
- YouTube has 800 million unique visitors per month; over four billion hours of video are watched per month.[13]

CONSUMERS DO MORE THAN LOOK FOR HEALTH INFORMATION ONLINE

A 2012 PricewaterhouseCoopers (PwC) report showed that one-third of consumers are using social media for health-related issues. Patients are not just seeking information about their diseases or symptoms, but increasingly they are looking for information about physicians and hospitals. Their research also showed that people choose community sites over industry-sponsored sites. When PwC tracked daily social media activity, it found consumers posted on community sites thousands of times versus hundreds of posts on company sites. Overall, community sites had 24 times more social media activity than industry-sponsored sites.[14]

U.S. consumers use social media in healthcare in many ways[5]:

- 25% of Internet users have watched an online video about health or medical issues.
- 23% of social network users, or 11% of all adults in the United States, have followed their friends' personal health experiences via social media.
- 34% of Internet users have read someone else's personal stories about health or medical issues on a website or blog.
- 27% of Internet users (20% of all adults) have tracked their diet, exercise routine, or some other health indicator online.
- 11% of social network site users, or 5% of all adults, have posted comments about health issues online.
- 14% of Internet users have signed up to receive alerts about health issues.
- 9% of social network site users (4% of all adults) have started or joined a health-related group on a social networking site.

The statistics above apply to the general population. But Internet users who have one or more chronic health conditions such as high blood pressure, diabetes, heart disease, or cancer are *even more likely* to read someone else's health stories online (37% vs. 31% of people who report no chronic health concerns), watch a health video (31% vs. 22%), or sign up to receive e-mail updates on medical topics (23% vs. 9%).[5]

Caregivers are also considerably more likely than other Internet users to use social network sites for following people's health updates (28%). Overall, one in five adult Internet users in the United States has used social media to find others who have similar health concerns. Social media connects people who share interests in all walks of life.

Susannah Fox, Associate Director of the Pew Internet & American Life Project, shares her perspective on what patients can expect from the intersection among healthcare, online media, and mobile technology:

"I don't know, but I can try to find out online" is now the default setting for a majority of people in the United States with health questions. "I know, and I want to share my knowledge" is the leading edge, as more people find ways to contribute to the online conversation about health.

Unfortunately, the other trend on the rise in the United States is the spread of chronic disease.

People living with chronic conditions and disability are disproportionately offline. These groups are the most likely to have significant health needs, but the least likely to have access to the most up-to-date information, such as drug recalls or new treatment options.

Two trends point a way forward, to a future that is not as bleak as it currently appears.

First, the "diagnosis difference." For the most part, Internet users with chronic disease are likely to be older and living in lower-income households—people who generally stay in the shallow end of the online activities pool, such as e-mail and search. But if we control for all other variables, living with chronic disease increases the likelihood that an Internet user will say that he or she works on a blog or contributes to an online discussion about health. People are learning from each other. And they say that these lessons are helping them to better manage their conditions.

Pew Internet has also identified a "mobile difference." If you hand someone a smartphone, he or she is more likely to become a contributor, a commenter, and a creator.

What will happen when the untapped knowledge of every patient, of every caregiver, of everyone who has something of value to share actually has the opportunity to share it? We are no longer tracking a linear trend of information retrieval, but rather a widening network trend, with everyone in the health system contributing to the conversation.

Susannah Fox
Associate Director
Pew Internet & American Life Project
Washington, DC
www.pewinternet.org

Kerri Morrone Sparling is a diabetes advocate who blogs at Six Until Me. In an interview with the blog ScienceRoll, she notes the profound power of community that social media brings[15]:

I've been living with Type 1 diabetes for 25 years. Part of what has helped me maintain good health is that feeling of community, and feeling like I'm not alone. Sometimes it can feel overwhelming, and there are things that your doctors can't give to you that can take that feeling away. They can't medicate that feeling of loneliness.

They can't medicate that feeling of, "I'm the only person with diabetes for miles."

What takes that away is knowing that I'm a part of a bigger community. There is a power to knowing that you're not alone. Sharing patient stories is crucial to emotional health. And good emotional health is crucial to maintaining good physical health.

My doctor can't sit across from me and say, "I know exactly what you're going through."

Unless she has diabetes, she can only guess. But my fellow patients, well, they know. And being part of a community that really understands is empowering.

Social media is also replacing face-to-face support groups.[5] Sherry Pagoto, PhD, Associate Professor of Medicine at the University of Massachusetts Medical School, describes how Twitter provides support for lifestyle interventions[16]:

As a clinical psychologist with research and clinical expertise in lifestyle interventions, I decided to take my skills to social media, via Twitter and a blog, as a way to disseminate my knowledge of evidence-based strategies for weight loss to the public. When I joined Twitter, I sought out other professionals doing the same, including dietitians, behaviorists, exercise physiologists, trainers, physicians, and the like. I was surprised to find them in such abundance and that many are purveyors of high-quality information. I also came across a subculture of Twitter users who use Twitter as a weight loss community.

I found more people than I can count whom I call real-life "biggest losers" because they have lost fairly substantial amounts of weight via lifestyle changes. They actively use Twitter and blogging to document their journey, share the secrets of their success, and connect with others who are on the same path. I love checking my Twitter stream and reading the chatter about morning workouts, friendly fitness challenges, and weight loss successes. I find myself congratulating strangers on their accomplishments and getting encouragement for my own.

> One day, I made a tweet "commitment" that I would be doing one abdominal plank each day (#plankaday) to overcome my dreadful history with core exercise. Over the months, 2000+ joined me. I was astonished. I don't know my followers personally, and I'm far from famous on Twitter. What it comes down to is the power of social networks for behavior change.
>
> Sherry Pagoto, PhD
> Associate Professor of Medicine
> University of Massachusetts Medical School
> Worcester, Massachusetts
> www.fudiet.com

Why should you, the healthcare provider, care about social media? The answer is simple: because that's where patients are going to be. Historically, they used the Web to look for information on their symptoms, their condition, or possible treatments, and they chose their doctors via word of mouth from friends and family or via their insurance company. But increasingly, as studies show, their health conversations are happening online. They want to know what it's like to get an MRI scan or to have diabetes. Most often, their personal physician cannot answer these questions because he or she may not have personal experience with the test or condition.

E-PATIENTS: A NEW BREED

The availability of online health information combined with social media channels has created a new generation of patients. We call them e-patients. They are empowered. They have a voice in their own care that they never had before.

Perhaps the most famous e-patient is Dave deBronkart, also known as e-Patient Dave. Back in 2006, Dave went to his doctor for a routine physical. He had some shoulder pain and went for an x-ray. The x-ray showed that the shoulder was fine, but his lung had multiple nodules. Further workup revealed that he had stage IV kidney cancer that had metastasized throughout his body.

In his TEDxMaastricht talk in 2011, Dave described what happened next[17]:

> My doctor prescribed a patient community, Acor.org, a network of cancer patients, of all amazing things. Very quickly they told me, "Kidney cancer is an uncommon disease. Get yourself to a specialist center. There is no cure, but there's something that sometimes works—it usually doesn't—called high-dosage interleukin. Most hospitals don't offer it, so they won't even tell you it exists. And don't let them give you anything else first. And by the way, here are four doctors

in your part of the United States who offer it and their phone numbers." How amazing is that? . . .

. . . The punch line is that a year and a half later, I was there when this magnificent young woman, my daughter, got married. And when she came down those steps, and it was just her and me for that moment, I was so glad that she didn't have to say to her mother, "I wish Dad could have been here."

Coincidentally, e-Patient Dave lives in Nashua, New Hampshire, just a few miles from where I live. And I've had the privilege of having breakfast with him several times, and our conversations are always fascinating because we approach the phenomenon of online patient engagement from different perspectives.

Even though deBronkart is a proponent of health information online, he still analyzes what he reads with a critical eye. He knows there is still a great deal of bad information on the Web, including information from companies trying to sell products or organizations pushing their own agendas.

Mark Britton, founder and CEO of the online legal rating site Avvo, which previously had a physician rating site before the latter was sold to HealthTap, says the Internet is where patients go today for pre-visit consultations[18]:

Patients are feeling empowered by the massive increase in plain-English, care-related information available on the Internet. On the other hand, they are feeling disempowered by the traditional healthcare system that is reducing their time in the system and thus their ability to get care-related information directly from their doctor.

The result? The Internet is the place where patients go for the pre-visit consultation. And love it or hate it, physicians must figure out how to participate in the online conversation because its use will only continue to grow. Patients can spend hours online researching their symptoms, looking at treatment photos and asking doctors questions about their condition. They can research a doctor's resumé, awards, publications and even possible misconduct. Occasional misinformation or not, this is far more patient-favorable compared to trying to cram the full-download into 13 minutes.

And, this should be physician-favorable as well. Yes, it is painful when the patient comes in with the Internet printout and they are horribly self-misdiagnosed; but that is the exception. The rule is that the patient comes in variably but incrementally smarter which speeds up the information exchange. The patient asks more-informed questions and the physician gives more-tailored advice.

IT'S STILL ABOUT THE DOCTOR-PATIENT RELATIONSHIP

Some doctors I talk to feel threatened by these newly empowered patients, saying that eventually, physicians will be marginalized.

I disagree.

No matter how much influence online health will have on patients, the core doctor-patient relationship will always remain paramount, according to Barbara Ficarra, RN, executive producer and host of the "Health in 30" radio show[19]:

> It's important for doctors, nurses and other health professionals to understand that Google, social media sites, health news and information sites and online patient community sites will not replace them. It's simply a tool that offers additional information, and it allows the conversation to get started between health provider and patient. Doctors, nurses and other health providers need to engage in the internet and social media platforms to help educate the health consumer. They have the power to provide accurate, reliable and truthful information. They should not [shy] away from the internet but embrace it and join forces with the health consumer. Partnering together is very useful and empowering.

> Additionally, the Internet will not change the underlying need for face to face interaction and engagement between doctor and patient.

In a worldwide survey, although the vast majority (93%) of people say they check their sources to make sure they're reputable, only 44% "always" check their sources; nearly half (49%) check them only "sometimes."[20]

According to a Pew Internet & American Life Project study, some patients are overwhelmed by the amount of health information online.[21] Others are frustrated or confused. And a minority are even frightened by what they find on the Web.

Physicians and other health professionals can and should be either a source of reputable information themselves or guide patients to better health websites. Physicians already use the Web to do their own searches. Studies found that 86% of physicians start their own health search with a search engine like Google or Yahoo.[22]

WHY SOCIAL MEDIA SHOULD BE IMPORTANT TO *YOU*

There are three reasons physicians should use social media to their advantage with patients:

1. ***Patients are going online to look not only for health information, but also to look for doctors, hospitals, and other healthcare entities.*** Today, instead of using the *Yellow Pages* to find nearby healthcare providers, they are probably going to

start by Googling their doctor's name. Every health professional needs to Google his or her name every week to see what comes up. This topic will be covered in detail in the next chapter.

2. ***Physicians can provide context to media health stories.*** When patients read health news in the newspaper or watch it on television, they really want to know what it means for them. Because of time and space constraints, there isn't enough commentary from health professionals in these stories. This is where social media comes in, because a social media platform, like a blog for instance, can provide health professionals with an outlet to write their commentary and give meaning to the stories patients read in the newspaper. It can be published immediately, meaning it can come out right after the news story appears and keep up with the pace of medical news.

3. ***Physicians can use social media to dispel myths.*** In addition to some health information on the Web being wrong, some of it is also dangerous. For example, despite the wealth of evidence that shows there is no connection between vaccines and autism, patients are still confused. A nationwide survey conducted several years ago asked, "Do vaccines cause autism?"[23] While 52% said "definitely no," this finding means that almost half of the people in this country aren't sure! Why does this happen? Part of the reason is that the Internet allows everyone to share their voice; it gives everyone a platform, which gives the illusion that every opinion is equal—and on many topics, that is not the case. On the Internet, people who took their last science course in high school are on equal footing with experts who have devoted their lives to the field. The Internet gives a platform to celebrities who can be factually inaccurate, yet they are tremendously influential. Every time there is media uproar about vaccines, vaccination rates fall for several years afterwards. Paul Offitt, MD, a leading physician and expert on vaccines, says, "it's much harder to unscare people than it is to scare them."[24] Celebrities and politicians can say whatever they want to plant seeds of doubt in patients' minds, but it's up to healthcare professionals to unscare patients in the exam room—that is a much harder job.

Healthcare professionals cannot afford to lose the PR battle online. If that happens, they risk losing their standing as healthcare authorities.

How can social media help? It gives health professionals an opportunity to tell their stories. If you turn on a daytime talk show, for instance, you may see a segment on vaccines and autism. On one side, there could be a doctor or public health official, who would have mountains of evidence on his or her side. But these experts usually speak in the language of numbers, data, and statistics. On the other side, there could be parents whose child has autism they think may have been associated with vaccines. They tell a powerful personal story, which could be tremendously persuasive in the arena of public opinion.

In a perspective piece from the *Journal of the American Medical Association*, physicians Zachary Meisel, MD, MPH, and Jason Karlawish, MD, note the power of the narrative.[25] "Scientific reports are genuinely dispassionate, characterless, and ahistorical," they write. "But their translation and dissemination should not be. Stories are an essential part of how individuals understand and use evidence."

In other words, stories put a human face on the evidence doctors rely on to teach and treat their patients. Social media provides an ideal stage to tell those stories.

Bryan Vartabedian, MD, is a Texas-based pediatric gastroenterologist who blogs at 33 Charts. He notes there are about 60,000 pediatricians in the United States. Imagine if every one of them wrote just one blog post a year talking about vaccines and autism. Just think how that flood of reputable health information would drown out the online presence of the vocal anti-vaccine minority.

Pediatrician Natasha Burgert, MD, tells a story of how her online presence helps build trust between her and her patients:

> "We are here because we read your blog," he said to me.
>
> While being interviewed by expectant parents, it is not uncommon for my blog to be mentioned. In fact, most new parents have subscribed to my blog before stepping foot in my office. I am pleased that my online reputation often precedes me.
>
> This encounter, however, seemed different. The father-to-be began discussing a specific post in detail. He listed key bullet points nearly verbatim. He commented that he had shared the post with his boss, due to its relevance to his line of work.
>
> He continued, "The article was very good. I compared it to similar posts by other pediatric bloggers in our area. And *this* post was the only one that got it right. That's why we are here. *You* got it right."
>
> His comment rang like a bell. Until that moment, I had thought of my online writing, curating, and sharing as a simple tool for patient families to augment healthcare decisions. After that meeting, however, it became clear that people were also using the information I posted as a measure of excellence, accuracy, and trustworthiness.
>
> My online reputation has become a mirror, reflecting my quality as a physician.
>
> Fortunately for me, discovering the importance of my online presence happened fairly early in my career. In turn, my efforts online have become very intentional and refined.

I continue to write, share, and curate online healthcare information. I add to my growing collection of child health information regularly. I promote other leaders in my field by sharing their amazing efforts, and I guide families to quality sources of health information to educate and to calm fears.

Ultimately, I carefully manage my online presence because I want to create a positive reflection of myself as a physician. This builds trust between my readers and me. And when trust has been gained, positive changes can be made.

Natasha Burgert, MD
Pediatrician
Kansas City, Missouri
http://kckidsdoc.com

HOW SIGNIFICANT ARE ONLINE DOCTOR REVIEWS?

Despite the increasing use of social media to track, discuss, and follow health-related issues, online doctor review sites are not yet in the mainstream of healthcare decision-making tools for most people.

According to the Pew Internet & American Life Project report of 2011, only 16% of Internet users have consulted a review site of physicians and other healthcare providers. However, it reports that caregivers and people with one or more chronic conditions are more likely to consult online doctor review sites—21% and 18%, respectively.[5] Pew data also show that only 4% have actually posted an online review of a doctor, but the PwC study puts this number a little higher, at 17%.[5,14] Any way you look at it, the impact of online physician ratings is increasing.

Doctors can take some comfort in the fact that most people still rely on medical information that they get from the real world, not in cyberspace. A 2011 PwC survey showed that 75% of patients still consult a physician if they have a health-related question (but 54% will consult online sources).[26] Gallup's Health and Healthcare Survey, released in late 2010, showed that 70% of consumers are confident about the accuracy of their doctor's advice and don't feel the need for a second opinion or additional research.[27]

Gallup's study also showed that older Americans are the most confident, with 85% of people over the age of 65 confident of their doctor's advice compared with 67% for those aged 50 to 64 and 65% of those under 50. Americans' evaluations of the quality of their own healthcare are among the most positive Gallup has found over the past decade, with 40% rating their healthcare as excellent, slightly higher than the previous high of 38% as well as the average of 34% over the past decade. A combined 82% rate their healthcare as either excellent or good, which is on par with previous years.[28]

When Sparling, the patient with diabetes mentioned earlier, suddenly had to switch doctors in the midst of her pregnancy, she turned to Google to do some quick research on her new physician:

> I didn't give much thought to the online reputation of any of my doctors until I was six months pregnant and was asked to switch OB/GYNs for delivery.
>
> My OB/GYN was moving to a different part of the practice, and the doctor the practice suggested as a replacement for her seemed kind and knowledgeable, and came highly recommended. But I was still wary. Who WAS this woman? I really liked my previous OB/GYN, and felt comfortable with her knowledge of high-risk pregnancies for women with long-standing type 1 diabetes. This new doctor was a mystery.
>
> So I consulted my dear friend Google to see what the Internet thought of this new doc.
>
> Online reviews are a curious thing, because most people don't log much time singing the praises of a product, service, or person. Usually, the Internet is crammed with people griping and complaining, serving as an outlet for people who might be frustrated or needing to vent. However, when I Googled my potential new doctor, I found a lot of information, mostly from other patients, that painted a much broader picture of what this new doctor was really like.
>
> What sealed the deal for me wasn't the CV-esque search return, listing the doctor's advanced degrees and academic achievements. Instead, I read dozens of blog posts, Facebook updates, and forum discussions about this doctor's bedside manner, and ability to remove some of the fear and anxiety about a diabetic pregnancy using her compassion and extensive medical knowledge. Hearing other patients say, "If I had to do this all over again, I'd want Dr. So-and-So by my side" made me feel comfortable switching doctors. The anecdotal experiences of others soothed my nerves and helped me transition doctors with confidence.
>
> Kerri Morrone Sparling
> Patient Advocate
> Coventry, Rhode Island
> http://sixuntilme.com

CAN YOU AFFORD TO IGNORE RATINGS AND SOCIAL MEDIA?

Although it might be comforting to know that only a small number of patients make decisions on their doctors based on online reviews, that mindset would be missing the point of social media. All of the data collected in recent surveys on the growth of social media show that this is where patients live today. Increasingly, it's where they find like-minded people, discuss common concerns, and share stories related to their health and well-being. Both the Pew and the PwC studies found that social media informs and influences over 40% of consumers today in their choice of a specific doctor.[5,14] Thus those physicians who play an integral role in the lives of their patients by being where they are—online—will come out ahead.

In fact, the 2012 PwC study also found that 61% of consumers are likely to trust information posted by healthcare providers.[14] That's much higher than the number (37%) who say they trust information provided by drug companies. These study findings are encouraging with respect to the fact that patients *still* rely on information provided by physicians and would continue to do so online.

Patients are also using social media to find and communicate their feelings about treatments; 24% of Internet users have consulted online reviews of particular drugs or medical treatments. In addition, 4% of Internet users have posted their experiences with a particular drug or medical treatment.[5]

Social media is not going away; it will continue to change and grow in ways that we can't even foresee today. Consider that Pinterest did not even exist three years ago, and now it is the third most popular site behind Facebook and YouTube.[29] Who's to say that the next social media break-out site won't be a health-related one?

Your hospitals are probably already using social media. However, U.S. hospitals are not leading the way in this area. Technology consulting firm CSC reports that hospitals in the Netherlands, Norway, Sweden, and the United Kingdom are moving the fastest toward embracing social media and using it for more than purely a marketing purpose. The United States is considered in the "mid range" of adoption according to the report. Within the United States, large academic and pediatric hospitals in metropolitan areas lead the way, with 42% of U.S. hospitals with more than 400 beds using social media, as compared with 15% of hospitals with fewer than 70 beds. In the category of teaching hospitals, 58% have adopted social media versus 16% in nonteaching hospitals.[30]

Mike Morrison is the Senior Public Affairs Officer and Social Media Specialist at Massachusetts General Hospital (MGH) in Boston, Massachusetts. Here's what he said when asked why it's important for hospitals to be involved with social media[31]:

To MGH, social media is essential to our mission. Our mission is to help people. If we know people are looking for help through social media channels, we should be there. For me, it's like us not having a website or telephone: how can we help if we're not using the same technology as our patients?

Your patients are definitely already using social media. Look at how internist Jordan Grumet, MD, learned this when he least expected it:

Lisa was a new patient who came in for a physical examination. She was a young-looking 30-something. She had a bag, which no doubt contained a computer, slung over her right shoulder. Her left hand clutched what appeared to be a few inches of computer printouts. I mentally rolled my eyes. It's not that I don't like my patients well informed, but I was just hoping to get through the physical without spending hours undoing whatever calamity her Internet search had produced.

My fears about Lisa faded quickly. She was respectful and to the point. The interview and exam flowed smoothly. Of course there were some issues here and there, but we talked through each without confrontation. She accepted my suggestions with minimal push back. I glanced at the printed pages on the desk as I finished my notes. They were just far enough away for me to be unable to make out the typed words.

As I waited for a moment for Lisa to ask any final questions, I couldn't help but wish that every new patient was like her: smart, organized, and ready to listen. When she assured me that there were no further questions, I got up to leave and reached for the doorknob. And that's when the feared bomb dropped.

Oh . . . Dr. Grumet, one more thing. I wanted to show you this!

I turned to find her thrusting the ream of papers toward me. I moved forward hesitantly and accepted the package with feigned indifference. I scanned the top of the page.

In My Humble Opinion

It was my blog. She had handed me a copy of my most recent blog posts. I looked up to find Lisa smiling.

I just wanted you to know why I chose you to be my doctor.

Jordan Grumet, MD
Internal Medicine Physician
Evanston, Illinois
http://jordan-inmyhumbleopinion.blogspot.com

Online reputation management has become a big concern for people in all walks of life. With the ever-increasing variety and use of social media today, managing one's online profile has never been more challenging or more important.

REVIEWS ARE MORE POSITIVE THAN YOU THINK

Despite the newness of physician rating websites in the United States, several studies have been performed to assess their value. The first formal study of physician rating websites was done in 2009 by Lagu et al. in Boston, and the results were published in the *Journal of General Internal Medicine* in 2010. The team studied 33 rating sites and searched for reviews of a random sample of 300 Boston physicians. As it happens, at that time, more than 70% of the physician sample did not have a review on any of the 33 sites! Their research turned up 190 reviews for 81 physicians, fairly evenly divided between generalists and specialists. Of those, 88% were positive, only 6% were negative, and 6% were neutral.[32]

A study of nearly 5000 online physician ratings using a somewhat different methodology was done in the fall of 2010 by researchers in California, Michigan, and Nebraska. They used Google Trends to identify the 10 most frequently visited online physician rating sites with user-generated content. They included only sites with more than 5000 daily unique visitors. Data from 4999 physician ratings across 23 specialties in 25 metropolitan areas were obtained. The researchers chose the cities with highest Internet usage and largest populations.[33]

The average rating according to their analysis was 77 for sites using a 100-point scale, 3.84 for sites using a 5-point scale, and 3.1 for sites with a 4-point scale. Furthermore, 61.5% of ratings on a 100-point scale were 75 or higher, while 57.74% had rating of 4 or higher on a 5-point scale, and 74% had ratings of 3 or higher on sites with a 4-point scale. In the final analysis, this study of nearly 5000 ratings across the 10 most popular rating websites showed that about two out of three patient reviews are favorable.[33]

A 2012 study by Gao et al. looked at 386,000 physician ratings on RateMDs from 2005 to 2010 and also found that the online reviews were generally very positive. The mean was 3.93 on a scale of 1 to 5. Nearly 50% scored a perfect (5 out of 5) rating. Only 12% scored below a 2 rating. The authors also found statistically significant correlations between the value of ratings and physician experience, board certification, education, and malpractice claims. While these data suggest a positive correlation between online ratings and quality measures, the impact is small. The average number of ratings per physician is still low, and ratings often reflect staff issues and punctuality more than clinical care.[34]

These studies help to dispel the myth that online reviews are generally done by disgruntled patients.

How can medical providers leverage these findings? Ask more patients to rate them online, good or bad, and let the proverbial chips fall where they may. That may seem counter-intuitive to most physicians, but chances are, the reviews will be better than most doctors would think. More reviews can not only help a physician's online reputation, but also make these sites more useful by populating them with more ratings. e-Patient Dave gives his opinion on the current state of online physician ratings:

> The primary consideration for me, in any reputation, online or off, is whose opinion I'm hearing and how they formed it. Their thought process, mental discipline, and personal values are fundamental. Without that, I have no idea if their rating would match mine.
>
> For that reason, I have no use for mere thumbs-up or -down ratings. I want Amazon-style written reviews, whose thinking and priorities I can assess. I also yearn for separate ratings for professional competence versus consumer friendliness, such as office hours, appointment lead time, time spent in the waiting room, clear billing, or online records.
>
> It's not just about patients getting what they want. The changes I foresee will make it easier for great providers to be recognized. Right now, if a hospital has an amazing transformation in medical errors, quality of care, or customer service it won't show up in the Hospital Consumer Assessment of Healthcare Providers and Systems (HCAHPS)—a survey that measures patients' perspectives on hospital care—for two years. That's a huge inhibitor to the normal market forces that reward good performers.
>
> We've solved this before. In eBay's early days, people said, "Who's going to buy online? You have no idea who you're buying from." But eBay added reputation, and today a mediocre reputation is death on that site.
>
> Even Amazon rates the raters.
>
> It's still early for online medical reputations. The tools are primitive and the culture still evolving. I expect it will mature, just as Amazon's and eBay's have. Until then, I won't put much stock in what I read, unless I'm sure who said it and what they were thinking.
>
> Dave deBronkart
> Patient Advocate
> Nashua, New Hampshire
> http://epatientdave.com

CAN ONLINE RATINGS BE COMPARED WITH CLINICAL OUTCOMES?

All of the studies described above point to the generally positive nature of online physician reviews. Many physicians wonder how ratings are tied to quality, or even if they can be. After all, there is great variability in the number of reviews and, in fact, in the number of patients or procedures performed among doctors. Add to that the subjective nature of the review process and the different metrics among review sites, and the picture gets even cloudier.

Doctors are often openly hostile to online ratings sites, with a few calling for their banishment, and most saying they add nothing of value to patient care.

But there is evidence in the medical literature that there are, indeed, positive correlations between patient satisfaction ratings and clinical outcomes.

A 2004 study by researchers at Press Ganey looked at inpatient ratings for patients hospitalized for five common conditions—heart attack, heart failure, stroke, pneumonia, and childbirth. Although patients with different conditions expressed different levels of satisfaction and had different care needs, this study found that patients who believed that their values and preferences were respected and that they had good emotional support from healthcare professionals had better outcomes. The researchers concluded that "good communication between patients and care providers drives positive patient experiences and compliance, which led to positive outcomes."[35]

A study conducted by Glickman et al. in 2010 examined the relationship between patient satisfaction and adherence to practice guidelines and outcomes for acute myocardial infarction. They used clinical data on 6467 patients treated at 25 U.S. hospitals, and cardiac patient satisfaction surveys from 3562 patients treated at the same hospitals during the same time period. Higher patient satisfaction scores were associated with lower inpatient mortality, even after controlling for a hospital's overall guideline adherence score.[36]

In the journal *BMJ Quality & Safety*, researchers from the Imperial College of London and the University of California-San Francisco looked at online posts from patients in the United Kingdom who received care at an acute general hospital in 2009 and 2010. The researchers looked at the relationship between online patient ratings on the National Health Service (NHS) Choices site, which was introduced in England in 2008, and paper-based surveys of patient experiences. The NHS site allows patients to post ratings on hospitals and practices, but not individual doctors. The researchers looked at nearly 10,000 Web-based ratings during 2009 and 2010. These ratings were compared with 68,500 responses to a formal inpatient survey during the same time period. This survey is done annually, using a random sample of patients, to gauge their opinions about the quality of care they received while in the hospital. Data on expected deaths, deaths from high-risk conditions, and emergency readmissions within a month of discharge were also collected.

An analysis showed that the unsolicited Web-based patient ratings correlated with the traditional survey measures of patient experience. Their responses matched on all four quality variables as well as on the percentage of patients willing to recommend the hospital to a friend (67.4%). They found that positive ratings correlated with lower overall mortality and readmission rates. In addition, hospitals that were rated cleaner by patients actually did have a 42% lower methicillin-resistant *Staphylococcus aureus* (MRSA) rate.[37]

A similar study in 2007 looked at the relationship between patient perception of hospital practices and infection rates in 87 Pennsylvania hospitals. The authors found that facilities with higher patient satisfaction scores on cleanliness, blood-draw skills, and nurse responsiveness tended to also have lower rates of infection and infection mortality.[38]

However, not all published studies reach positive conclusions about patient ratings as they relate to clinical outcomes. A 2012 study from the *Archives of Internal Medicine* gives credence to some physicians' fears that obtaining good ratings means giving in to patients' demands. According to the study, compared with the least-satisfied patients, those who were most satisfied with their healthcare were taking more prescription medications, had more doctor's office visits, and were more likely to have had one or more hospital stays, despite the fact that they were in better overall physical and mental health. Also, despite the greater attention and all those prescription drugs they got, the highly satisfied patients were more likely to die in a few years after taking the survey than were those who pronounced themselves least satisfied with their physicians' medical care.[39]

As an emergency physician who blogs pseudo-anonymously at *Emergency Physicians Monthly* bluntly puts it, "'High satisfaction' with a health care facility means that you're more likely to be admitted, you're more likely to pay more for your care, and you're more likely to be discharged in a body bag."[40]

Not only are satisfied patients more likely to die, they cost more: Overall, the most satisfied patients incurred 8.8% more healthcare expenditures than did the least satisfied and spent some 9.1% more on prescription drugs than did the least satisfied.[39]

While we wait for more studies to conclusively decide whether or not online ratings improve patient care, reviewing doctors on the Web is a phenomenon that isn't going to simply disappear. Already, 27% of consumers post reviews of restaurants, hotels, or products, according to PwC data.[14] It's only a matter of time before the majority will want to share their reviews of their doctors and hospitals online as well.

LARGE-SCALE INITIATIVES USING PATIENT RATINGS

Patient satisfaction ratings figure prominently in several large-scale initiatives that have the potential to affect both the reputation and bottom line of every medical practice. The federal government has taken some important steps in this direction through the policies of the Centers for Medicare & Medicaid Services (CMS). The venerable ratings organization Consumer Reports is now also more heavily involved in the healthcare field with its recent release of a report on primary care practices in Massachusetts.

In what may be the largest initiative yet on transparency, the CMS announced in late 2011 that it will make its claim data available to the public.[41] As a result of this ruling, insurers, institutions, and employers will have access to all billing data from Medicare and will be able to create online tools to assist patients in making informed decisions about their healthcare. While CMS has rated hospitals and nursing homes for several years, this is the first time it has focused on individual physicians.

In addition, for the last few years, CMS has done surveys of a random sample of patients discharged from the hospital to measure their perspectives on the care they received. Patient ratings from HCAHPS are available on the CMS website via a link for "Hospital Compare."[42]

A similar survey aimed at measuring patients' experience with physicians is being tested now. The Clinician and Group Consumer Assessment of Health Providers and Systems, or CGCAHPS, questionnaire seeks patients' reviews of care given by physicians in the office. The CMS created a "Physician Compare" website in 2011.[43] Beginning in 2013, it will include data collected through the Physician Quality Reporting System (PQRS). The patient ratings of physicians could be added to the website. The data also become part of a CMS plan to establish a "value modifier" that provides for variable payments to hospitals and physicians based on quality of care.

In October 2012, CMS began adjusting payments to hospitals based on the new metrics.[44] Individual physicians have also started receiving reports from CMS showing how the quality and cost of care they provided to their Medicare patients in 2010 compares with that of their peers. Right now, these report cards are being used only in Nebraska, Missouri, Iowa, and Kansas. The Physician Feedback/Value-Based Modifier Program is part of a program that will move from a volume-based fee-for-service system to one based on value, as mandated by the new Affordable Care Act. Although the payment modification won't start until 2015, CMS has started measuring physician performance as of January 1, 2013.[45]

Patient satisfaction data are a key component of the new metrics, the idea being that patients who have a better experience will have better outcomes. There is a great deal of debate over that belief, as well as other related issues, such as "safety net hospitals," but those health policy debates are outside the scope of this book. *What's important here is that 30% of a hospital's quality score will be determined by patient ratings of the hospital!* Payment models for physicians will change, too, and will also likely include patient satisfaction ratings for measurement of quality.

Medicare insures more patients than any other single insurer and is a major payer for most medical practices. As the population ages, this trend will only intensify. Furthermore, where Medicare goes, private insurers are sure to follow. Many insurers already collect patient reviews or license information from one of the major rating sites as a service to their members. Whether those ratings ultimately affect physician payments is not known, but is certainly within the realm of possibility.

In June 2012, Consumer Reports, the nonprofit organization most known for its ratings service of everything from cars to refrigerators, issued a report on primary care practices in Massachusetts. The ratings were compiled in partnership with Massachusetts Health Quality Partners (MHQP), a coalition of physicians, hospitals, government agencies, consumers and insurers, and researchers.[46]

MHQP has been conducting and reporting patient experience surveys since 2006. Consumer Reports used data from a 2011 survey to produce a special supplement to its magazine that was distributed to subscribers and available on newsstands throughout Massachusetts.

The report, called "How Does Your Doctor Compare?," is also available for anyone to read online at www.mhqp.org. It covers 329 physician group practices and 158 pediatric practices, with ratings completed by more than 64,000 Massachusetts residents. The results are presented in Consumer Reports iconic layout of symbols. Survey questions addressed communication, coordination of care, how well the doctors got to know their patients, patients' experience with office staff, wellness advice, and pediatric care.

The ratings for each doctor in a practice were pooled into one overall score per question, and reported on a 4-point scale. Most practices earned top ratings in several measures, and nearly all practices lacked in some areas. Only 13 of the 329 adult practices surveyed obtained a top score on all five ratings categories. However, the report notes that "overall, scores for physician practices in Massachusetts have been on the upswing" since MHQP first started doing the surveys six years ago. MHQP's goal is to provide both patients and physicians with information that can be used to improve the quality of care and outcomes.

It's worth noting that, despite the breadth of this new effort, not all physicians are included in the ratings. Only practices with three or more physicians are included.

The Consumer Reports/MHQP initiative was funded by the Robert Wood Johnson Foundation through its Aligning Forces for Quality program, which is aimed at improving quality of care in 16 communities across the United States. These organizations believe that the transparency offered by the patient experience ratings provides opportunities for doctors and patients to work together to build strong partnerships and achieve better outcomes. Thus the trend to seek and distribute patient ratings of physicians seems likely to continue.

WORKING TOWARD A HEALTHCARE PARTNERSHIP

When doctors face patients who come to their visits with printouts from health information sites on the Web, they have two choices. They can roll their eyes and tell these patients not to go online, as I know some of my colleagues do. Or they can embrace it, and realize that no matter what they do or what they think, it's going to happen anyway.

As we noted at the beginning of this chapter, patients are not only looking for health information on Google, but also on social networks like Facebook. These sites are popular with patients who, according to the Pew Internet & American Life Project, generally gravitate toward user-generated information. It's no wonder that 65% of adults online use social networking sites, with patients reading other people's commentaries or experiences with a particular test or treatment.[47] But can these communities substitute for advice from a qualified health professional?

A 2011 study from Harvard Medical School, which looked at 15 of the largest Facebook diabetes communities and analyzed close to 700 "wall" posts, provided some insight. Most of the comments provided support among diabetics and included strategy tips, personal advice, and emotional outreach. But more than a quarter of posts were promotional in nature, advertising non-FDA-approved products of questionable efficacy or safety.[48] So although social networks have definite value in connecting patients, the information needs to be viewed with a critical eye.

With only 7% of doctors e-mailing their patients,[49] let alone engaging them on blogs, Twitter, or Facebook, the medical establishment needs to realize the influence of the Internet and social media on patients.

Pediatrician Burgert calls for an evolution in the doctor-patient relationship in today's digital age:

> Navigating health online information is a learning process for all of us. If we don't listen to each other, we don't learn.

If patients and doctors can have open dialog about information found online—good and bad—we can take care of patients better. And that is more than Dr. Google could ever do alone.[50]

Guiding patients to better online sources of medical information should be a new physician responsibility for the digital age. Not only should doctors expect and be receptive to questions patients ask from Web research, they need to proactively engage patients online in order to dispel falsehoods and guide them to legitimate sites. Until then, patients should be vigilant about checking the source of what they read on the Web to make sure it comes from a reputable institution—such as a hospital, medical school, or government agency.

The economic incentives, coupled with changing demographics and readily available online tools to disseminate information, mean that there is no going back. A more transparent healthcare system is here to stay, and the use of online physician rating sites is likely to grow as well. What's missing from the current online rating system would be enhanced by both the qualitative and quantitative data that will soon be available on every practicing physician. The visibility of quality data can provide incentives to doctors to deliver the highest quality of care, which, in turn, leads to better outcomes and more positive online reviews. Government and private Web initiatives are complementary efforts that change the game of medical practice.

The Internet, and social media in particular, has fundamentally changed the doctor-patient relationship by breaking down the information barriers traditionally separating patients from their health professionals. How both parties navigate this new paradigm will determine how much the Web and social networks will benefit patients.

Like it or not, as more information becomes available about doctors and hospitals online, information about you and your practice will be on the Web. Your level of activity on social media is a decision for you and your practice, but managing your reputation is critical. We'll explore ways to research and manage your online reputation in the chapters that follow. ▪▪

REFERENCES

1. Fox S, Duggan M. Health Online. Pew Internet & American Life Project. 2013; http://pewinternet.org/Reports/2013/Health-online.aspx.

2. Social media. Wikipedia, The Free Encyclopedia. http://en.wikipedia.org/w/index.php?title=Social_media&oldid=521345659. Accessed November 4, 2012.

3. Social media—Definition and More from the *Free Merriam-Webster Dictionary*. www.merriam-webster.com/dictionary/socialmedia. Accessed October 29, 2012.

4. PAFP Big 3: Primary Care & Social Media. http://issuu.com/pafppublications/docs/pafpsocialmediaguide1?mode=window&backgroundColor=#222222. Accessed October 29, 2012.

5. Fox S, Jones S. The Social Life of Health Information. Pew Internet & American Life Project. 2011; www.pewinternet.org/Reports/2009/8-The-Social-Life-of-Health-Information/02-A-Shifting-Landscape/1-Americans-are-tapping-into-a-widening-network-of-both-online-and-offline-sources. aspx. Accessed October 29, 2012.

6. Jansen J. Online Product Research. 2010; http://pewinternet.org/Press-Releases/2010/Online-Product-Research.aspx.

7. Selingo J. The bell is tolling for the beeper. *New York Times*. April 11, 2002; www.nytimes. com/2002/04/11/technology/the-bell-is-tolling-for-the-beeper.html?pagewanted=all&src=pm. Accessed October 29, 2012.

8. One Billion People on Facebook. Facebook Newsroom. October 4, 2012; http://newsroom.fb.com/ News/One-Billion-People-on-Facebook-1c9.aspx. Accessed November 4, 2012.

9. What is Twitter? Twitter for Business. https://business.twitter.com/basics/what-is-twitter. Accessed November 4, 2012.

10. Elliott A-M. YouTube Facts: 10 Things You May Not Have Known. Mashable. 2011; http://mashable. com/2011/02/19/youtube-facts. Accessed November 4, 2012.

11. Health Care Social Media: Getting Executives on Board. Healthcare Association of New York State. April 2012; www.hanys.org/communications/social-media/assets/docs/health_care_social_media. pdf. Accessed November 1, 2012.

12. Bennett S. How Do People Spend Their Time Online? [INFOGRAPHIC]. AllTwitter. May 7, 2012; www.mediabistro.com/alltwitter/online-tim e_b22186. Accessed November 1, 2012.

13. YouTube Statistics. www.youtube.com/t/press_statistics.

14. Social Media "Likes" Healthcare. PwC Healthcare Institute. 2012; http://pwchealth.com/cgi-local/ hregister.cgi/reg/health-care-social-media-report.pdf. Accessed November 3, 2012.

15. Sparling KM. Why an e-patient should blog! ScienceRoll. December 18, 2011; http://scienceroll. com/2011/12/18/kerri-morrone-sparling-why-an-e-patient-should-blog.

16. Pagato S. Refer patients to Twitter for weight loss. KevinMD.com. March 8, 2012; www.kevinmd. com/blog/2012/03/refer-patients-twitter-weight-loss.html. Accessed October 29, 2012.

17. deBronkart D. Meet e-patient Dave. TED. June 2011; www.ted.com/talks/dave_debronkart_ meet_e_patient_dave.html.

18. Britton M. The Internet is where patients go for pre-visit consultations. KevinMD.com. January 26, 2012; www.kevinmd.com/blog/2012/01/internet-patients-previsit-consultations.html.

19. Ficarra B. Social media starts the patient dialogue with doctors and nurses. KevinMD.com. May 10, 2010; www.kevinmd.com/blog/2010/05/social-media-starts-patient-dialogue-doctors-nurses.html.

20. BUPA Health Pulse 2011 International Healthcare Survey. 2011; www.bupa.com/media/288798/ bupa_health_pulse_report_2011.pdf.

21. Fox S. Pew Internet & American Life Project Online Health Search 2006. 2006; www.pewinternet. org/Reports/2006/Online-Health-Search-2006/01-Summary-of-Findings.aspx.

22. Parekh N, Mayer J, Rojowsky N. Connecting with Physicians Online: Searching for Answers. November 2009; www.fdasm.com/docs/Connecting with Physicians Online Webinar Deck-- final.pdf.

23. Vaccine-Autism Link: Sound Science or Fraud? Harris Interactive. January 20, 2011; www.harris interactive.com/newsroom/pressreleases/tabid/446/mid/1506/articleid/674/ctl/readcustom%20 default/default.aspx.

24. Parikh R. Make Anti-Vaccine Parents Pay Higher Premiums. CNN.com. January 21, 2011; www. cnn.com/2011/OPINION/01/20/parikh.childhood.immunizations/index.html. Accessed November 5, 2012.

25. Meisel ZF, Karlawish J. Narrative vs evidence-based medicine: and, not or. *JAMA*. 2011; 306:2022-2023.

26. Top Health Industry Issues of 2011. PricewaterhouseCoopers; www.pwc.com/us/en/health-industries/publications/top-health-industry-issues-of-2011.jhtml.

27. Most Americans Take Doctor's Advice Without Second Opinion. Gallup. 2010; www.gallup.com/poll/145025/Americans-Doctor-Advice-Without-Second-Opinion.aspx. Accessed November 1, 2012.

28. Americans' Ratings of Own Healthcare Quality Remain High. Gallup. 2010; www.gallup.com/poll/144869/americans-ratings-own-healthcare-quality-remain-high.aspx. Accessed November 5, 2012.

29. The 2012 Digital Marketer: Benchmark and Trend Report. Experian Marketing Services. 2012.

30. Should Healthcare Organizations Use Social Medi a: A Global Update. CSC. http://assets1.csc.com/health_services/downloads/CSC_Should_Healthcare_Organizations_Use_Social_Media_A_Global_Update.pdf. Accessed November 3, 2012.

31. Gualtieri L. Social Media Strategy at Massachusetts General Hospital (MGH). KevinMD.com. March 9, 2011: www.kevinmd.com/blog/2011/03/social-media-strategy-massachusetts-general-hospital-mgh.html.

32. Lagu T, Hannon NS, Rothberg MB, Lindenauer PK. Patients' evaluations of health care providers in the era of social networking: an analysis of physician-rating websites. *J Gen Intern Med*. 2010;25:942-946.

33. Kadry B, Chu LF, Kadry B, Gammas D, Macario A. Analysis of 4999 online physician ratings indicates that most patients give physicians a favorable rating. *J Med Internet Res*. 2011;13(4):e95.

34. Gao GG, McCullough JS, Agarwal R, Jha AK. A changing landscape of physician quality reporting: analysis of patients' online ratings of their physicians over a 5-year period. *J Med Internet Res*. 2012;14(1):e38.

35. Gesell SB, Wolosin RJ. Inpatients' ratings of care in 5 common clinical conditions. *Qual Manag Health Care*. 2004;13:222-227.

36. Glickman SW, Boulding W, Manary M, et al. Patient satisfaction and its relationship with clinical quality and inpatient mortality in acute myocardial infarction. *Circ Cardiovasc Qual Outcomes*. 2010;3:188-195.

37. Greaves F, Pape UJ, King D, et al. Associations between Internet-based patient ratings and conventional surveys of patient experience in the English NHS: an observational study. *BMJ Qual Saf*. 2012;21:600-605.

38. Trucano M, Kaldenburg D. The Relationship between Patient Perceptions of Hospital Practices and facility Infection Rates: Evidence from Pennsylvania Hospitals. *Patient Safety & Quality Healthcare*. Online Feature 2007; www.psqh.com/enews/0807feature.html. Accessed November 4, 2012.

39. Fenton JJ, Jerant AF, Bertakis KD, Franks P. The cost of satisfaction: a national study of patient satisfaction, health care utilization, expenditures, and mortality. *Arch Intern Med*. 2012;172:405-411.

40. WhiteCoat's Call Room: A Death Knell for Press Ganey? Emergency Physicians Monthly. February 13, 2012; www.epmonthly.com/whitecoat/2012/02/a-death-knell-for-press-ganey. Accessed November 4, 2012.

41. Centers for Medicare & Medicaid Services. Medicare Gives Employers, Consumers Information to Make Better Health Care Choices. 2011; www.cms.gov/apps/media/press/release.asp?Counter =4206&intNumPerPage=1000&.

42. Centers for Medicare & Medicaid Services. Hospital HCAHPS. 2012; www.cms.gov/Medicare/
Quality-Initiatives-Patient-Assessment-Instruments/HospitalQualityInits/HospitalHCAHPS.
html. Accessed November 5, 2012.

43. Centers for Medicare & Medicaid Services. Physician Compare Fact Sheet. May 2012; www.cms.
gov/Outreach-and-Education/Medicare-Learning-Network-MLN/MLNProducts/Downloads/
PhysicianReview-ICN904144.pdf. Accessed November 5, 2012.

44. Centers for Medicare & Medicaid Services. Hospital Value-Based Purchasing. www.cms.gov/
Medicare/Quality-Initiatives-Patient-Assessment-Instruments/hospital-value-based-purchasing.

45. Centers for Medicare & Medicaid Services. Physician Value-based Payment Modifier and the
Physician Feedback Program. www.ntocc.org/Portals/0/PDF/Attachments/PublicPolicyUpdates/
FSV-MPFS-2013-NPRM-20120706.pdf.

46. Consumer Reports/MHQP. *How Does Your Doctor Compare?* July 2012; http://c354183.r83.cf1.
rackcdn.com/MHQP%20Consumer%20Reports%20Insert%202012.pdf.

47. Madden M, Zickuhr K. 65% of Online Adults Use Social Networking Sites. August 26, 2011; http://
pewinternet.org/Reports/2011/Social-Networking-Sites.aspx.

48. Greene JA, Choudhry NK, Kilabuk E, Shrank WH. Online social networking by patients with diabetes: a qualitative evaluation of communication with Facebook. *J Gen Intern Med*. 2011;26:287-292.

49. Boukus ER, Grossman JM, O'Malley AS. Physicians Slow to E-mail Routinely with Patients. Center
for Studying Health System Change. October 2010; www.hschange.com/CONTENT/1156.

50. Burgert N. Do You Google Your Child's Symptoms? KC Kids Doc. February 7, 2011; http://kckids
doc.com/do-you-google-your-childs-symptoms.html.

"Best keep yourself clean and bright; you are the window through which you see the world."

—George Bernard Shaw

CHAPTER 2

Your Online Identity Today

HOW PATIENTS FIND DOCTORS TODAY

When new patients come to my exam room, the first thing I normally ask them is how they found me. When I started practicing medicine 10 years ago, patients would say they found me either through the *Yellow Pages* or a newspaper ad, or from calling the local hospital. But more and more frequently, patients are saying that they found me through the Internet.

Searching the Internet is so popular that the word "Google" has now officially become a verb. The vast majority of us search for information on the Internet. This trend in my practice is consistent with data from the Pew Internet & American Life Project. Its most recent survey on search engine use, released in February 2012, showed that 91% of adult Internet users employ search engines, up from 84% in the previous survey done in 2004. Every day, 59% of us are searching the Web, as compared with 30% who did online searches each day in 2004. Even though more and more people are turning to social media to interact with others on the Web, they are *also* searching more often. Not surprisingly, adults younger than 50 and those with more education and higher incomes search more frequently than others.[1]

In Chapter 1, several studies were described regarding the impact of the Internet on consumers' search for health information and, increasingly, on their choice of providers. For most people, finding a doctor is a task done locally. Thus it's interesting to note how the search for medical care stacks up against searches people do for other types of local businesses.

In the first quarter of 2012, search engine optimization consulting firm BrightLocal sought to determine what types of local businesses people look for online and the importance of reputation on those searches. Local consumers in the United States, Canada, and United Kingdom were surveyed. Data were collected on almost 3000 consumers and compared with a similar study done in 2010 with U.S./UK participants. This study was not specific to healthcare but produced results that shed light on trends in online searches and reviews.

Not surprisingly, the most searched type of business was restaurant/café (57% vs. 37% in 2010). But this study also showed that consumers' search for doctors and dentists is one of the top-growing categories of search, with 27% of consumers searching vs. 21% just two years earlier. This finding is notable given that many types of businesses (for example, hair salons, specialty shops) saw their search numbers go *down* in the same time period. The researchers concluded that consumers are more focused today on essential rather than nonessential services; healthcare is clearly an essential service for most people.

Responses to the question about online reviews showed even more dramatic results—21% of consumers said they now read online reviews for doctors and dentists, nearly double the number (11%) from just two years earlier. In fact, it was one of only two categories that had an increase in the usage of online reviews as part of the search process; many types of businesses, including hotels, actually had a decrease in the number of people who read their online reviews.[2]

Can patients reliably choose a good doctor online? Inevitably, some will. But there are some good reasons why consumers should be wary of the information they find online about doctors. Many doctors are not comfortable being visible online. So if you do not have a blog or a social media profile, what shows up when a patient Googles you most likely will be something from an online rating site. Figure 2.1 is an example.

WHY YOUR ONLINE IDENTITY IS IMPORTANT

The first step in determining your online reputation is simple—Google yourself. But before you do, you may want to read the rest of this book . . . and brace yourself. You may find mixed results, some positive and some negative reviews. Most likely, the results of your Google search will be inconclusive, as Figure 2.1 illustrates. Most of the rating sites found during a Google search will contain basic data, such as where you went to medical school, years in practice, and the names of hospitals where you work. On some of the sites, that is all the information you will find. There may be a couple of reviews from patients, but on many sites, there will be none at all. Then why waste time looking, you may ask? There are several reasons why doing a Google search now will pay off in the future:

1. ***Establishing a positive presence.*** As we've seen with data reported from various studies and surveys, consumer use of the Internet to not only find but to comment on their experiences with healthcare is growing. If you do not have many ratings now, consider yourself lucky that you're able to get in on the ground floor in establishing a positive online presence and cultivating positive reviews from your patients. Even your current patients may be watching!

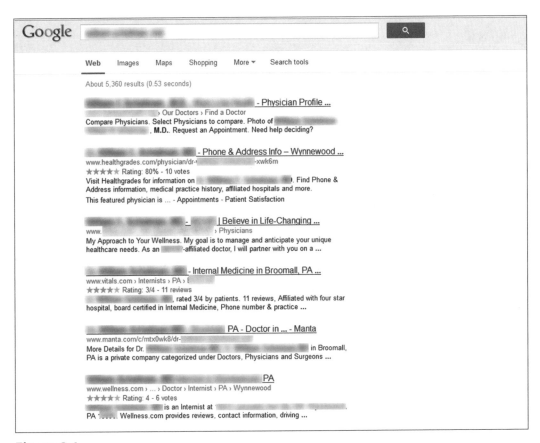

Figure 2.1

2. ***Correcting errors and out-of-date information.*** You may find errors in some of your listings and can correct them so potential patients know where to find you. Most rating sites allow physicians to manage their basic data. We'll cover this in more detail in Chapter 5. An old address or telephone number can cost you. If you have moved to a new practice but the group you were previously with still exists, potential patients who call your old phone number will probably be offered an appointment with a doctor in that group. Your former practice is not likely to pass on your new contact information!

3. ***Having no reputation is as bad as having a negative reputation.*** Next year or the year after, when potential patients do a search and find several physicians' profiles that meet their criteria for specialty or geography, do you really want yours to be the one with no information about your practice? Increasingly, patients will be making decisions based on other people's opinions. A straightforward and positive online presence could boost your business now, as more patients find you and decide to make an appointment with you based on what they've read.

4. ***Knowledge is power.*** No one wants their weaknesses broadcast to the whole world. Understandably, many healthcare professionals are nervous about the transparency

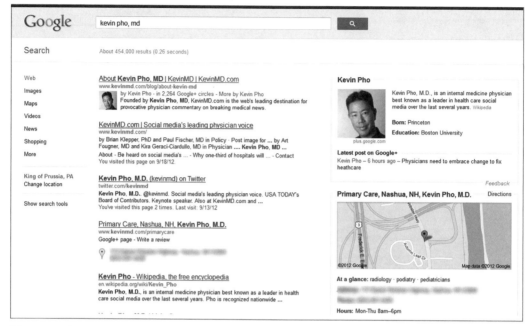

Figure 2.2

brought about by social media, especially the trend toward online reviewing by patients. But think about the kinds of Google searches you do. Perhaps you've used TripAdvisor to plan a vacation or read hotel reviews. You've most likely Googled an unfamiliar restaurant to find reviews of what other people thought of it. How many of those hotels or restaurants have had 100% positive ratings? Probably none. Feedback can be healthy, allowing you to discover ways to improve patients' experiences with all aspects of your practice.

5. ***Claiming your identity.*** One fact of life in our increasingly small and interactive world is that there are no names that are truly unique to one person. No matter how unusual you think your name might be, chances are there is at least one other person somewhere in the world with the same name and with an Internet presence.

When I Googled myself a few years back, numerous ads appeared, promising readers a "detailed background report" or "profile" of me. Among the search results was information about my practice, whether I was board certified and had any lawsuits against me, and reviews from online doctor rating sites. Thankfully, most reviews were favorable, but some were not. But when patients type my name into a search box, they also see my many online presences, ranging from my blog to various social media profiles—and most importantly, these results are listed *first*. Figure 2.2 is the first page of my search results.

Internist Vineet Arora, MD, tells a story of what happened the first time she Googled herself. See what she did about it:

My online reputation was not something I had ever thought of until I had a bad one. When someone would Google my name, he or she would find the top hits referred to my exact namesake, Vineet Arora, an ophthalmologist in Ontario, Canada. This would not be so terrible, except that most of the links were accompanied by a headline like "Ophthalmologist accused of blinding patients."

Needless to say, that really concerned me.

Would people think I was that guy? My name and even professional identity were associated with this other person. What's worse is that my own faculty profile at the University of Chicago was not coming up high in the search. So at that moment, I decided to generate my own online content.

The first thing I did was set up a LinkedIn account as a landing page for myself that included a list of my positions. I will confess that I was afraid of being too "out there" at first, so I kept my LinkedIn page pretty bare-bones. While I had started embracing Twitter, I was still experimenting and purposely did not link my Twitter to my formal name "Vineet Arora" but instead used "Vinny Arora," a more personal name my friends know me as. Well, there was really no reason to worry.

Twitter has changed my life. Through Twitter, I have made contact with a vast network of individuals interested in improving medical education and healthcare. Through Twitter, I have received numerous speaking invitations, media inquiries, and job offers. I even have a funded grant with an individual I have not yet met in person! I have also made many friends, some of whom I have actually met.

I link all my social media accounts to my LinkedIn page. I also created a Google profile and a very cool about.me page to aggregate Web content related to my work.

Controlling my online reputation allows me to control what people say about me, too. For example, when I give talks, I simply send my Google profile bio, as opposed to having someone reinvent the wheel from my CV.

I share my story with trainees so that they not only become familiar with their online reputation, but also take control of it. Even if they are not ready to dive fully into social media, setting up a LinkedIn page is an easy first step to building an online reputation.

Because I see patients only when they are hospitalized in an urban academic center that cares for an underserved, diverse population, my patients don't likely know who I am until they meet me. But these days, the minute you hear about someone you don't know, what do you do? You Google them. So I would not be surprised if that is what some of my patients do, and certainly more will do so in the future.

In this day and age, because your online reputation is often your first impression, it better be a good one.

Vineet Arora, MD
Internal Medicine Physician
Associate Program Director, Internal Medicine Residency Program
Pritzker School of Medicine, University of Chicago
Chicago, Illinois
http://futuredocsblog.com

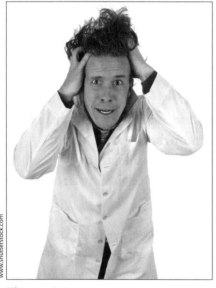

www.shutterstock.com

Figure 2.3

But whenever I discuss online physician ratings with other healthcare providers, the mood in the room changes. A sense of anxiety emerges (see Figure 2.3), as most physicians have not been trained to deal with being reviewed online.

Most physicians I talk to say their greatest fear is Googling their name and seeing a negative review from one of these sites. What if, when you Google yourself, you were to find comments like these:

"Going to this dermatologist was a waste of time and money."

"What a mistake. This man has the bedside manner of someone from the Amazon."

These comments were taken from real reviews at a physician rating site. It's obviously not how you want patients to find you on the Web.

Despite the risks to your online reputation that bad reviews can bring, many physicians still don't see the value of both social media and the time it takes to develop a strong online reputation. If you want to determine the impact of social media on your practice, you can use a metric every business uses to measure the impact of its investments of time and money: the return on investment (ROI). Simply ask new patients how they found you. You may find that a growing percentage of new patients coming to your office are there because of information they found about you online.

Over the past year, I've kept track of how new patients found me. Ten percent to 15% say it's because of my online presence. Howard Luks, MD, an orthopedic surgeon in New York who also has a strong social media profile online, estimates his numbers to be between 15% and 17%.[3]

And finally, the research firm YouGov found that 57% of consumers said that a social media connection was likely to have a strong impact on their hospital choice.[3]

Social media's ROI is starting to be quantified and will surely grow as more patients go online.

GETTING TO KNOW YOU

Even if a patient has been referred to your practice by another physician or by a family member or trusted friend, chances are he or she will turn to the Internet to learn more about you before scheduling an appointment. Searching online is now the default whenever anyone simply wants more information about any topic or person. Similarly, patients choosing you because you're in their health insurance network doesn't mean they are coming to you blindly either. They may have gotten your name from an insurance company site, but they will likely also look you up online.

Patients who've explored your practice online may also be more comfortable with you, because they may feel as though they already know you. They may be more willing to share their concerns because they've seen a video of you or read an article or interview about you. In addition, because they made a conscious decision to come to YOU (perhaps even selected you from among several choices), they may be more receptive to your instructions. Not only might this enhanced comfort level make the relationship between you and your patient stronger, it could minimize the chance that the patient will go elsewhere after the initial visit. Isn't this a more productive way to engage with patients?

John Mandrola, MD, is a cardiologist who isn't afraid to use his online presence to share his opinion. See the opportunities that arise because of it:

> **My online reputation is a matter of great humor at home and at work.**
>
> **One of my partners sometimes hollers down the hall, "Here comes the great Dr. John M."**

That's really funny because my family and other doctors know me as nothing special. I don't write scholarly papers, I did not attend an Ivy League school, and rarely do I get on local TV.

But because I have an online presence, a voice, I have something. A following. A tribe. A presence. A lectern. A class. My son calls it a postage-stamped-sized country. Even he admits that it's growing.

Why is this remarkable? So many doctors, and many of my generation, are scared to have any presence online. A journalist friend recently wrote to me that my writing had grown and was greatly improved. He was impressed by my "willingness to put yourself out there in front of the whole world while you learn your craft."

Maybe it's this lack of fear to put oneself out there that strikes folks like my partner.

To me, it's stunning how much people are drawn to real-world opinions. When I was shopping around for opinions on whether I should have a controversial shoulder surgery, I would have loved to have come across a plain-speaking doctor-expert. That's what I am looking to give people: a non-think-tank, real-world voice. Of course, I want my voice to be respected and serious, but it has to be less filtered. It has to be real. It has to be me.

A year or so ago, I would have said most patients in Kentucky had no idea that I write a blog or use Twitter. But that's changing. More and more, patients tell me they have read my blog.

I think about patients when I hit "publish" or tweet. I don't want them to think that I am unprofessional. That said, I do go out of my way, and I take every opportunity, to remind them that doctors are human. This comes up when they "like to complain" about a medical mishap. I emphasize that humans practice medicine.

I manage my online reputation the same way I manage my real-life reputation. I try to be honest, right-minded, and compassionate. I don't see a difference between online and real-life reputations.

John Mandrola, MD
Cardiac Electrophysiologist
Louisville, Kentucky
www.drjohnm.org

NOT EVERYONE IS CONVINCED THAT DOCTORS NEED A STRONG ONLINE PRESENCE

Many physicians say they do not want a strong online presence or to participate professionally with social media. To discover some reasons behind these opinions, family physician Ted Eytan, MD, went to Sermo, a closed, online community of physicians who can post under anonymous or pseudo-anonymous handles. He asked this community, "Why isn't my doctor using social networks?" Here is a sample of responses:

I agree . . . that social media tools have enormous potential to help an integrated healthcare system fulfill its purpose, especially in a fully accountable, coordinated care delivery system. Based on my years in self-employed private practice, in the currently fragmented, transaction-oriented care system, I don't think these interactive tools are as well suited to the purposes of self-employed physicians or those working in independent physician group practices.

The problem is we are stretched to the limit with junk work (not patient or medical problems of patients but the impact of third-party systems) . . . I cannot afford to have endless Twitter conversations with patients. The distraction is bad for patient care or office functioning.[4]

And consider what family physician Dike Drummond, MD, says about social media:

If you are a clinician who is paid by your patient's insurance company for the services you provide, I challenge any social media consultant to show you how a Facebook post or Twitter tweet produces any additional income for you.

Remember, no one pays you to login and post on Facebook. You would have to be posting something that actually causes more patients to come into the office where you can see them and charge for your services.

Before you do anything on social media, I encourage you to understand exactly how you generate a return on that investment of time and energy.

If you are the typical doctor in the typical medical practice, there is no business case for social media, there is no ROI, and the additional workload and expectations could worsen the amount of stress you are under. That's three strikes by my reckoning.

So the next time a "guru" of social media tells you the five sites you should be on, you can say, "Thanks, but no thanks," and get back to taking good care of your patients and spending time with your family instead.[5]

Of course, I disagree with these assessments, but there is clearly some entrenched skepticism that needs to be overcome when it comes to doctors using social media. Time will tell who's right.

YOUR CAREER ALSO DEPENDS ON YOUR ONLINE REPUTATION

Googling people is so commonplace now that most recruiters and human resources personnel use it regularly to get information on potential employees. So patients may not be the only people Googling you! If you are actively seeking a new job or looking to move to a new area and have networked with colleagues or contacted hospitals and medical groups regarding employment or affiliation, you should expect these people to Google you as well.

Joseph Kim, MD, is a physician-executive who blogs at Non-Clinical Medical Jobs, Careers, and Opportunities. Here he describes how social media can help doctors find job opportunities online:

> Many physicians intentionally choose to avoid online social networking websites like LinkedIn, Facebook, and Twitter. Physicians want to maintain their privacy, and they don't want patients "finding" them on these public sites.
>
> If you're thinking about a career transition or if you're looking for non-clinical jobs that may provide supplemental income, it is very important to expand your social network by engaging others on social networking websites. There are ways you can do this while still maintaining your privacy.
>
> Physicians are finding job opportunities by networking with other physicians online. Online social networking is also a valuable tool for those who want to spend some time conducting informational interviews. You may find interesting people who may be willing to provide you with information about how they reached that point in their career. You may find physicians working in industry who would be willing to speak with you about day-to-day responsibilities, tasks, challenges, and opportunities. You may even find physicians who are willing to introduce you to hiring managers and other executives in their own organizations.
>
> If you're thinking about a career transition, don't be afraid to meet new people online. You may find the perfect opportunity by expanding your network and by learning about companies and career opportunities that you didn't even know existed.

To start, I would encourage you to join LinkedIn. Then join Facebook and adjust your privacy settings based on your personal preferences.

Joseph Kim, MD
Physician Executive
Newtown, Pennsylvania
www.nonclinicaljobs.com

FIRST, DO NO HARM; SECOND, GET AN ONLINE PROFILE

The online ratings system is only as good as the information it contains. Garbage in, garbage out. Given the complexity of medicine and the vagaries of consumer opinion, it will never be a perfect system.

Rating sites vary widely, with many that use their own scale to determine ratings. Some sites allow anonymous posting of comments, while others require that consumers use their own names. You should take the time to create a profile on the reputable sites. Twelve of the major rating sites are profiled in Chapter 5. These sites rank highly in search engines and have been identified by researchers as the most important for physicians and other healthcare professionals. Although they differ widely in scope, demographics, and rating criteria, all of the rating sites listed allow physicians to set up their own profile free of charge and manage the information displayed. Note that the basic information that they have about you and your practice may not be correct! Many of the rating sites license information from commercially available databases that may contain outdated or otherwise inaccurate data. This information is then carried over to your profile on the rating site, where it becomes visible to consumers searching for healthcare providers. Thus it's essential to not only claim your profile but also to keep it updated. You can create profile information and apply it consistently across all of the rating sites even though each site has somewhat different functionality.

In the anecdote below, Seattle-based psychiatrist Maria Yang, MD, has used her Web presence not only to shape her online identity, but also as an opportunity to meet others through the Web that have influenced her professionally:

There is already a lot of information about you, as a physician, on the Internet. This can include where you work, where you trained, and any opinions that people—patients or otherwise—may have about you. Someone else is already defining who you are and what you do. This may come as a surprise to those physicians who are unaware that they have online reputations.

Thus creating and maintaining your own corner of the Internet gives you the power to shape your online identity.

While some physicians may argue that online reputations are trivial, remember that patients search the Internet to learn about their symptoms and medical conditions. Sometimes they read information that is accurate. Sometimes it is wrong. This information can influence how they move forward with their healthcare. This same process occurs when patients seek information about their doctors.

Physicians rightly worry about boundary issues and having an online presence. Some fear that patients may use social media to seek medical advice, attention, or services. To be clear, that risk is there. In my experience of having an online presence for over 10 years, my patients have never contacted me through my website with requests for medical advice, extra attention, etc. During office visits, however, my patients have offered support and compliments about my writing online. The vast majority of people respect professional boundaries and do not cross them.

My online presence has introduced me to a variety of people—some in medicine, many who are not, all of whom have interacted with the healthcare system—who have helped me become a better physician. They have provided unique perspectives, asked good questions, and shared interesting information. This has been the greatest reward of having an online presence.

Maria Yang, MD
Psychiatrist
Seattle, Washington
www.inwhiteink.com

WHICH SEARCH ENGINES SHOULD YOU USE?

There are hundreds of search engines on the Internet at any time. New search engines are being developed all the time, and older ones may fall by the wayside. It pays to try to stay current with search engines. Remember AltaVista? It was widely considered the number 1 search engine in the days before Google. Ever heard of Axis? Yahoo! recently released it as an iOS app and a desktop browser version. There are more than 30 general search engines and many more of a specialty nature.

Google is by far the most popular search engine used today; most people start their searches there. The Pew study found that 83% of Web searchers use Google more often than they use other search engines. Yahoo! came in a distant second, with just 6%. Here again, we see big differences between search engines used in 2012 versus those used in 2004 when 47% used Google, and 26% favored Yahoo!.[1]

Internet analytics company comScore captures over one trillion interactions monthly. Its September 2012 search engine rankings also showed that Google leads, but with a somewhat different market share of 66.7%, followed by Microsoft's Bing at 15.9% and Yahoo! at 12.2%.[6]

A study published in the *Journal of Medical Internet Research* in March 2012 looked at the search engines consumers often use to obtain medical information. In that study, the authors named Google, Yahoo!, Bing, and Ask.com as the four major search engines for health and medical information.[7]

Google is where you want to start your own search to determine your online reputation. You should search your name in several ways (i.e., full name with middle initial, name called by, nickname, even common misspellings).

You might start by simply putting your name into the search box. When you do a simple search on your name or practice name, the first result may be the website of your practice or group. But as the example in Figure 2.1 shows, unless you are active in social media, the next results are likely to be a variety of third-party review sites.

After you get search results for your name, look at the comments on review sites (if any). What are patients saying about your staff? Do any themes emerge from looking over reviews from different rating sites? Many doctors tell me that they have never Googled themselves. If you are among them, you may be surprised at the information you find. You probably already have an online presence—but did you create it or did others?

Jeff Livingston, MD, an obstetrician-gynecologist in Texas, implores doctors to "Google thyselves" to find out:

> Have you ever Googled yourself or your practice? Did you know that you have an ever growing online reputation? Whether you know it or not, doctors have an online presence. Everything you do professionally creates a digital footprint. If you are involved in social media then you are contributing to your online reputation. If not, your online reputation is being written for you. There is a conversation taking place about you online, but unfortunately you may not be included in it.[8]

Academic emergency physician Nicholas Genes, MD, PhD, does just that. He describes how his Google footprint has given him advantages over his colleagues:

As an emergency physician, I don't rely on my online reputation to attract patients to my practice. But I recognize the importance of maintaining a professional Web and social media presence; and as an academic researcher, I want potential collaborators to be able to easily find me, review my work, and interact with me.

People who search for me on Google, after reading one of my articles or hearing a presentation, will find either my landing page (www.nickgenes. com) or my blog—both of which allow easy communication with me and showcase some of my work. I have received writing, editing, reviewing, speaking, and job offers through my landing page's contact form.

For instance, in response to a blog post (http://blogborygmi.blogspot. com/2010/12/they-might-be-giants.html), the wife of my favorite medical school professor contacted me to let me know how much she appreciated my noting his passing and my praise for their book.

Compare that with my efforts to reach some colleagues in which case I land on something like a Healthgrades ratings page, which may show—if I'm lucky—a snail-mail hospital address that may not even be current. I recently revised a chapter in a major emergency medicine textbook, and the previous edition's author is entirely unreachable through Web searches, which is hard to imagine in this day and age.

Beyond accessibility, however, I want my online presence to be professional, while still reflecting some of my personality. In addition to peer-reviewed publications and contact info, www.nickgenes.com has my tweets, blog posts, and some photos, as well as songs I've chosen to "scrobble" to the website (via www.last.fm).

I once walked into a job interview, and my interviewer was actually playing the music I'd been listening to a few days before. We began the interview by discussing music, my travel photos, and my recent blog posts, which is a great way to start if you've chosen your songs, pictures, and words with some care.

Nicholas Genes, MD, PhD
Emergency Physician
Assistant Professor of Emergency Medicine
Mount Sinai School of Medicine
New York, New York
www.nickgenes.com ▪

REFERENCES

1. Pew Internet & American Life Project. Search Engine Use 2012. March 9, 2012; http://pewinternet. org/Reports/2012/Search-Engine-Use-2012.aspx. Accessed November 5, 2012.

2. Anderson M. Local Consumer Review Survey 2012: Part 2. Search Engine Land. May 7, 2012; http:// searchengineland.com/local-consumer-review-survey-2012-part-2-120321. Accessed November 3, 2012.

3. Health Care Association of New York State. Health Care Social Media: Getting Executives on Board. April 2012; www.hanys.org/communications/social-media/assets/docs/health_care_social_media. pdf.

4. Eytan T. Discussing social media with physicians on Sermo. KevinMD.com. June 8, 2011; www. kevinmd.com/blog/2011/06/discussing-social-media-physicians-sermo.html. Accessed November 5, 2012.

5. Drummond D. Why social media may not be worth it for doctors. KevinMD.com. April 30, 2012; www.kevinmd.com/blog/2012/04/social-media-worth-doctors.html. Accessed November 3, 2012.

6. comScore Releases September 2012 U.S. Search Engine Rankings. comScore, Inc. October 11, 2012; www.comscore.com/Insights/Press_Releases/2012/10/comScore_Releases_September_2012_U.S._ Search_Engine_Rankings. Accessed November 5, 2012.

7. Wang L, Wang J, Wang M, et al. Using Internet search engines to obtain medical information: a comparative study. *J Med Internet Res.* 2012;14(3):e74.

8. Livingston J. Doctor, Google thyself. KevinMD.com. December 8, 2011; www.kevinmd.com/ blog/2011/12/doctor-google-thyself.html. Accessed November 3, 2012.

"Do not go where the path may lead, go instead where there is no path and leave a trail."

—Ralph Waldo Emerson

CHAPTER 3

Defining Your Online Identity Through Social Media

SOCIAL MEDIA CAN BE A POWERFUL TOOL

For managing the way you and your practice appear in search engines, a social media offense is a good defense. By proactively creating content, you can manage your online reputation and drive down any negative reviews that may exist. But social media can be so much more. As some of the stories in Chapters 1 and 2 demonstrate, it offers a powerful way for you to educate and engage with patients, and ultimately, achieve better outcomes. More transparency can lead to improved patient safety. Social media can also connect you with other professionals and keep you current with developments in your field. All of these issues affect your reputation and the reputation of the medical profession as a whole. Now is the time for all healthcare providers to harness the power of social media as patients have.

Here is a memorable example of how one patient used social media to seize control and make a difference in his own care.

In 2009, John Schumann, MD, an internist currently practicing in Oklahoma, contacted me to tell me about a friend of his, who happened to be a Harvard law professor. He had been having profuse, nightly fevers without a clear cause.

In her *New York Times* column profiling the case, physician Lisa Sanders, MD, further described the situation this patient was facing:

The fevers started a week after he returned from a conference in Switzerland, the patient told [his physician, Dr. Andrew] Modest. They only came at night, but they came every night. First the fever and then hours later he would break out in a heavy sweat. Sometimes it was so bad that he had to change his pajamas and sheets. He had a tickly kind of cough, too. Other than that, he had no pain. The patient said he had lost 15 pounds over the past month, but assumed that was because he started a new diet.

The doctor found nothing out of the ordinary. The patient had no fever, although his temperature had gone up to nearly 102 the night before. His heart rate and blood pressure were normal. So was everything else.

The patient had fever for four weeks and lost a good deal of weight, which the doctor thought could not be attributed to the minor dietary changes. Was this an infection? Maybe, although he didn't look sick. Was it some sort of autoimmune disease like lupus? Or was it some sort of cancer? Any of these were possible.[1]

At that point, an abdominal CT scan was ordered, which showed a mass in the patient's liver.

The patient was then admitted to the hospital for further workup. The medical team focused on the liver mass, wondering if it was a hemangioma—a non-cancerous liver tumor—although this condition does not typically cause fevers. Perhaps it was an abscess, but after sticking a long needle into the liver, no abscess was found. The medical team was at a diagnostic standstill.

Schumann was telling me about this case, when he dropped a bombshell. This patient was *live blogging his hospital stay.*

The patient had a laptop computer at his bedside; and whenever he would talk with a consulting physician or received the results of a lab test, he would type it up and post it on his blog, hoping someone would read it and chime in on the case. The term "crowdsourcing" means to tap into the collective intelligence of the public at large. In this case, the patient was crowdsourcing his diagnosis.

Amazing! I had never heard of such a thing, so I posted this patient's story on my site as it was unfolding, knowing that many physicians who saw it on my site would go over to the patient's site. In this way, the patient wouldn't just get second and third opinions, but he could get hundreds of physicians' opinions.

I'll let the patient himself describe what happened next, from one of his blogs posted while in the hospital:

> The blog produced some amazingly helpful comments from people and doctors at large, including references to two discrete academic journal articles—one from a Korean medical journal from 1994! Thanks to the Net I had a copy on my PC and then e-faxed to the nurse's station on my floor in a matter of minutes. In the meantime, over the course of today, additional results have come back to help narrow the diagnosis in a properly documentable and formal way—one that's converging, it seems, to the obscure Korean article.[2]

HERE ARE SOME OF THE MANY THINGS YOU CAN DO WITH SOCIAL MEDIA

1. Improve the visibility of your practice
2. Increase patient traffic, increase revenue, and build your practice
3. Act as a filter—refer patients to the best sites
4. Actively communicate with and positively influence the lives of patients even when they're not in the office for medical care
5. Create and post information that you use repeatedly to save time in the long run
6. Forge deeper connections with your patients
7. Be a preferred provider—anecdotally, we know that some patients prefer a doctor who is active on the Internet (or at least has a presence there) to one who is not
8. Build a referral network
9. Increase loyalty to your practice
10. Follow leaders in your field, stay up to date, and share with colleagues
11. Become a strong voice on healthcare issues
12. Promote your brand by creating meaningful content
13. Gain recognition
14. Create information that enhances your online reputation
15. Save money on traditional advertising, which can be reduced or eliminated with social media visibility

That article from the Korean medical journal showed that hemangiomas, those benign liver tumors, above a certain size could indeed cause fevers every night.

As a result, the law professor underwent a complicated surgical procedure to remove the liver mass, which indeed turned out to be a giant hemangioma. After the surgery, the patient's fevers resolved.

For me, this fascinating case was the most profound example of a patient using social media to have a proactive voice in his own care. It's time for healthcare professionals to use social media's power to have a similar impact on their professional lives. Let me show you the possibilities.

CURATE, CONNECT, AND MAKE A DIFFERENCE

Over the years, I haven't used social media just to connect with patients. I have also met a number of fascinating healthcare professionals from around the world. I have not only connected with them, I have learned from them as well. For example, one of the biggest problems I have with the Internet is that there is just *too much information*—too many articles to sift through. Wouldn't it be nice to have thought leaders in any area of medicine who can pick and choose the best articles for you?

That's what I use a real-time social media platform like Twitter for. On Twitter, you can put together a list of thought leaders and not only read what they have to say—briefly—but also click through to read a full article that they are sharing. In so doing, I use social media to curate and filter the Web. It is one of the most powerful ways to stay current in medicine.

Indeed, more doctors are learning through social media. A September 2012 study from the *Journal of Medical Internet Research* found that 85% of oncologists and primary care physicians used social media at least once a week to explore health information, and 58% perceived social media to be good way to consume current, high-quality information.[3]

One of the thought leaders I've connected with online is Paul Levy, former CEO of Beth Israel Deaconess Medical Center in Boston, Massachusetts, and one of the few hospital CEOs who had an active blog. As CEO, he wrote about issues most hospitals won't even talk about, such as the infection rate in the intensive care unit as well as medical mistakes that some of the physicians on his staff had made.

One story on his blog involved a patient who went into the hospital to undergo foot surgery. When the patient woke up in the recovery room after the procedure, he looked at the bandages on his foot and asked his doctor one question: why are the bandages on my left foot instead of my right? To that doctor's horror, he at that moment realized that he had operated on the wrong foot.

When Levy heard this story, he didn't punish the doctor. He didn't try to sweep the incident under the rug. Instead, he wrote about it on his blog. Why would he do that? Because he believed that "real time public disclosure can be mutually instructive."[4] He didn't want just his hospital staff to learn from this mistake. He wanted other hospitals to learn as well, so that they wouldn't make the same mistake. Levy also strongly believes that transparency is a strong motivator to improve patient safety. What could be more transparent than social media platforms, such as blogs?

I have also learned from patients using social media. Their perspectives are important because many healthcare professionals don't see medical situations from the perspective of a patient. Kerri Morrone Sparling is a patient with type 1 diabetes who posted about her wedding and how she handled her insulin pump as well as her diabetes on that important day.[5]

If this patient came to me for advice for her wedding day, I probably wouldn't know what to say because I don't have direct experience with this condition. But on her blog, Sparling wrote about asking her seamstress to sew a pouch in her gown for her insulin pump, as well as a little compartment in the holder for her bouquet where she could store candy in case her blood sugar got low during the festivities.

Not only is it valuable for patients to share their experiences with each other, but it's also valuable for healthcare providers as well. The next time a patient with a similar situation comes to my office, I'll know what to say and how to guide her.

THE NEWS MEDIA DON'T PAINT A POSITIVE PICTURE

I find it discouraging when I talk to students and residents who tell me that their administrators are not very interested in social media. They're being told: don't go online, don't use Twitter, be careful with Facebook. Fourth-year students tell me they have to delete their Facebook profiles because they are scared of what residency directors will find. Unfortunately, it's true that much of the media coverage of healthcare social media is negative.

Imagine opening a newspaper and reading this headline: *Doctor fired over Facebook posts.*

This story appeared in a Boston newspaper last year. An emergency department physician at a Rhode Island hospital posted interesting case studies on her Facebook page. Although she did not identify the patients by name, the details of one trauma case were unusual enough that someone who knew the patient and saw the post recognized the patient. Even though the doctor removed the post after the controversy began, she still lost her hospital privileges and was sanctioned by the Rhode Island state medical board.[6]

Instead of banning social media, we all need to encourage, educate, and promote the right way for healthcare professionals to use it. We need to be as professional on the Web as we are face-to-face with a patient, and we always need to be aware of HIPAA rules. When you use any form of social media, ask yourself before you hit the send button: If I were in a crowded hospital elevator and I said aloud what I just wrote for a social media network, would that be OK? If the answer is no, don't post it! Information on the Internet spreads quickly, and you could get into trouble like the doctor in Rhode Island if you are not careful.

Furthermore, we need to send a more positive message when it comes to social media and healthcare. Brian McGowan, PhD, an education technology consultant, surveyed doctors' attitudes when it came to social media. Of those surveyed, 20% said social media was a bad idea, 30% thought it was great, and the remaining 50% were in the "movable middle."

According to McGowan, if more studies and news stories highlighted its positive side, perhaps that 50% of physicians in the middle could be swayed toward using social media.[7]

ESTABLISHING A SOCIAL MEDIA STRATEGY TO CREATE YOUR OWN CONTENT

Medical practices are diverse, and social media offers a great many choices for you to become involved in the digital world. But you need to develop a strategy that will guide you in this endeavor. Your goals and objectives may be quite different from those of your colleague in another specialty. A primary care physician may need to use different social media than an anesthesiologist, for instance. Your patient population can guide you to some degree. If you see mostly older patients, Twitter might not be the best place to engage them. But did you know that the fastest growing segment of Facebook's membership is women over the age of 55?[8]

Think about your objectives as you read the descriptions and guidelines that are featured in Chapter 4. Will social media be a component of your marketing strategy? Will you use it to advance your career? Do you just want to stay informed and protect your reputation? How much time are you prepared to spend on social media? Do you have staff that can help you implement your social media strategy?

Social media can and should be tailored to each individual practitioner's goals, personality, and strengths. Experts say personal blogs, websites, and personal social media pages all tend to rank high in search engine results. Studies have shown that 90% of people doing searches do not go past the first page of search results, and 99% do not go past the second page. Internet marketing firm Optify looked at Google search results from December 2010 and found that the top three search results got 60% of the clicks with an average 37% click-through rate for ranking at the top of the first page.[9] These results show that ranking not only on the first page of Google search results, but close to the top of those results, is valuable. Thus it makes sense that one of the best ways to secure a good online reputation is to manage the content that appears on the first page or two of a search for you.

There are two avenues that you can use to own your name online, and thus own your online reputation. As described in Chapter 2, the simplest is to claim your profile on major review sites and make sure the information in it is correct and kept up to date.

The other avenue involves creating your own content. Chapter 4 is devoted to the major social media channels—LinkedIn, Facebook, YouTube, Twitter, blogs, and Google. Yes, Google—it's not just a search engine. Using these social media tools, you can create your own brand identity and define your online reputation by generating content. You have no control over what other people say about you, but you have total control of the content you create about yourself and your practice. Chapter 4 presents guidelines on being proactive with social media and creating your digital footprint, along with stories from physicians currently using these tools.

LURKING AS A FIRST STEP

Dr. Westby Fisher, who blogs at Dr. Wes (http://drwes.blogspot.com), recently suggested a strategy for doctors reluctant to take part in social media. He advised them to "lurk" instead of "engaging" with patients and peers . . . at least as a first step toward having a social media presence. He advised doctors to open an account on some of the social media channels, then "follow a group of people with common backgrounds and interests to yours, and *don't say or type a thing.* Just listen."[10]

By creating an account, you are reserving your name on that social media platform and can decide later how you want to interact with the site. Lurking allows you to not only observe but also get accustomed to the processes used in contributing to it. Fisher believes that:

> . . . even the most skeptical of physicians will see how these services can bring ideas and insights to them that they simply would never have had any other way . . . Just learning how to listen to the social media conversation not only provides an opportunity to participate in the medium IF (and only if) the doctor desires, but permits an instantaneous opportunity to raise one's voice to affect change when it's really needed.[10]

As you develop your overall social media strategy, lurking may become your due diligence phase.

THREE PHYSICIAN SOCIAL MEDIA SUCCESS STORIES

Cardiologist Kevin Campbell, MD, recounts how his online presence positively impacts his professional development and how he became recognized by the Heart Rhythm Society as a social media authority for his specialty:

> **For me, online reputation is extremely important. The Internet is timeless, and cyber footprints are permanent. Social media, in particular, has provided me with many opportunities to expand my practice and educate my patients.**

> **For example, I was travelling to the University of Colorado in Denver to conduct a symposium on "Prevention of Sudden Cardiac Death in Women."**

I tweeted from the airport that I was excited to speak about the subject and that my goal was to impact the lives of under-served and under-treated patients. Within minutes, I received a tweeted response from a physician group in my hometown that I had not previously received referrals from. The group asked that I reach out to them and conduct a similar symposium in my hometown.

Once back in town, I followed up with the senior partners in the group that I had connected with via Twitter. Now they are a major source of my referrals. Were it not for my Internet presence, I may have never been fortunate enough to have interacted with the new group and have had the opportunity to impact the lives of the patients that the group has referred.

Beyond patient care opportunities, my online reputation has also impacted my career and afforded me with wonderful professional opportunities. For example, because of my prolific blogging and significant Twitter presence, I was recognized by the Heart Rhythm Society and asked to develop an educational course on social media in medicine for the society's 2013 annual educational sessions. Additionally, due to my social media presence and frequent blogging, I was featured in a national publication, *EP Lab Digest,* and have since become a regular contributor to both the online and print editions.

My online footprint is important to my professional development, my career, and my patients. I take great care to protect my online reputation and to continually work to expand my Internet presence every single day.

Kevin Campbell, MD
Cardiac Electrophysiologist
Raleigh, North Carolina
www.drkevincampbellmd.com

Obstetrician-gynecologist Jeff Livingston, MD, has learned he needs to go where his patients are. At first, that was MySpace. But since then, they have migrated to Facebook and other social media sites:

Back in the day, there was only MySpace. No one used the term "social media." Facebook and Twitter existed only as vague ideas. My 15-year-old daughter taught me the power of online patient engagement. She changed the course of my practice and the way I approach patient care.

I was a new doctor just starting private practice and trying to make a name for myself in my local community. I was volunteering time at the local high schools giving lectures on preventing unplanned teen pregnancy and sexually transmitted disease.

One night, I was sitting at home discussing that day's presentation with my family. My daughter was using the computer. Looking over her shoulder, I was curious as to what she was doing. She was working on her MySpace page. At that point, I had only heard of MySpace and had no real idea of what it was or why anyone would use it. My daughter suggested that I create a MySpace page for myself and then make it available the next time I spoke at a high school. She helped me create the page that night.

At the end of my next lecture, I nervously put up my MySpace page. There was audible giggling in the audience but before I drove back to the office I started getting friend requests and messages from teenagers all over Irving, Texas, asking serious questions about sexually transmitted disease and pregnancy prevention. These were questions young people would never have been comfortable asking out loud in front of an audience. They may not have been comfortable asking privately face-to-face in a doctor's office either.

I recognized that while I was striving to make a difference in these young people's lives, I was trying to communicate with them in traditional ways. But the truth is, these young people lived online—they lived on MySpace. To connect with them, I had to go where the audience was. From there, our social media strategy was born. A light bulb went off in my head. Within a year, hundreds of young people were connecting with me online getting answers to their medical concerns and building a stronger, more personal doctor-patient relationship.

I learned the value of expanding the doctor-patient relationship beyond the four walls of the office. I also learned that the more patients were educated, the easier my job in the office became. Our use of social media turned a traditionally challenging demographic of lower socioeconomic, urban teenagers into educated healthcare consumers.

Since then, MacArthur OB/GYN has expanded its use of Internet technology. We have a robust website, a patient portal, an electronic health records system, three active blogs, and a presence in social media channels like Facebook, Twitter, HealthTap, and YouTube. We know that a patient who is educated and engaged in her own health makes the care we provide better and our jobs as healthcare providers easier. We understand that technology can expand the doctor-patient relationship.

Jeff Livingston, MD
Obstetrician-Gynecologist
Irving, Texas
http://macobgyn.com

And finally, family physician Davis Liu, MD, notes how social media gave him an opportunity to contribute an authentic, authoritative voice to the national healthcare conversation:

In the fall of 2007, my book publicist recommended I begin posting things online to build my "platform" for my upcoming self-published book. Unlike other more established authors, I did not have connections or a built-in brand like a radio show or newspaper column, which is often necessary for a successful launch.

So I started my blog with a few posts. Like my book, my posts reflected my thoughts about what patients needed to know about the American healthcare system, the latest updates in medical news, and changes in health policy. Unlike my book, however, posting online allowed immediate feedback and commentary about the latest news.

Over time, my posts made it to websites, like KevinMD.com, that had large readerships. My opinions were now being critiqued both positively and negatively nearly in real-time. This feedback was incredibly valuable in shaping and sharpening my own points of view.

From my brief experiences, three principles have emerged.

First, to be most authentic and credible, doctors should post under their own name. By publishing with your name, you are fully accountable for what you post or respond to. As a result, you will add thoughtful dialog to move the conversation forward. As a consequence, you are building a reputation, yours.

Second, whether you believe it or not, as a result of what you write, forward, or tweet, your true voice will come through. Others will challenge your perspectives. Learn from their insights, and challenge them as well. Over time, it will be increasingly clear what your voice is and what you stand for. Unless you actively try, it's hard to consistently create a completely different persona. When I've met people who I've connected with only online, the vast majority have said, "I feel like I know you." What you say truly reflects the essence of who you are.

Finally, expect to be engaged at a level that will reinvigorate your love of medicine. Doctors are teachers, healers, and among the most trusted individuals in society. We have knowledge and expertise, which is not valued by the current healthcare system. By being online, we are free from the time constraints of the office visit. We can leverage our time better because our thoughts and perspectives are online for anyone to see and view both today and in the future. Our voice can be heard in a way simply not possible just a few years ago.

As our country struggles with the challenge of how to make our healthcare system more affordable, more accessible, and of higher quality, the content and discussions we create online will be incredibly important to ensure that we as a society make the right choices and are always focused on the sacred doctor-patient relationship.

This is why we became doctors.

This is why doctors must be online.

This is why you need to be online.

Davis Liu, MD
Family Physician
Sacramento, California
www.davisliumd.com

REFERENCES

1. Sanders L. The heat of the night. *New York Times Magazine*. September 10, 2010; www.nytimes.com/2010/09/12/magazine/12FOB-diagnosis-t.html?_r=2&. Accessed November 5, 2012.

2. Zittrain J. The Future of Zittrain Has Not Been Stopped. The Future of the Internet—And How to Stop It blog. March 15, 2010; http://futureoftheinternet.org/jz-update. Accessed November 5, 2012.

3. McGowan BS, Wasko M, Vartabedian BS, et al. Understanding the factors that influence the adoption and meaningful use of social media by physicians to share medical information. *J Med Internet Res*. 2012;14(5):e117.

4. Levy P. We saved one person's life. Can we keep it going? Not Running a Hospital blog. February 16, 2007; http://runningahospital.blogspot.com/2007/02/we-saved-one-persons-life-can-we-keep.html. Accessed November 5, 2012.

5. Sparling KM. Diabetes on My Wedding Day. Six Until Me blog. June 3, 2008; http://sixuntilme. com/blog2/2008/06/diabetes_on_my_wedding_day.html. Accessed November 5, 2012.

6. Conaboy C. R.I. doctor fired over Facebook posts. Boston.com. April 19, 2011; www.boston.com/ news/health/blog/2011/04/ri_doctor_repri.html. Accessed November 5, 2012.

7. Dolan P. Doctors tell how they use social media as professional watercooler. *American Medical News*. October 22, 2012; www.ama-assn.org/amednews/2012/10/22/bisc1022.htm. Accessed November 5, 2012.

8. Hertz J. 5 Tips for Expanding Your Hospital Facility's Social Media Presence. The Comfort & Style Connection Blog. September 1, 2012; www.comfortstyleconnection.com/2012/09/01/5-tips-for-expanding-your-hospital-facility's-social-media-presence. Accessed November 5, 2012.

9. Unger T. The Changing Face of SERPs—Organic Click Through Rate. Optify. March 1, 2011; www. optify.net/search-marketing/organic-click-through-rate. Accessed November 5, 2012.

10. Fisher W. What Social Media Can Bring to the Physician Skeptic. Dr. Wes Blog. April 7, 2012; http:// drwes.blogspot.com/2012/04/what-social-media-can-bring-to.html. Accessed November 5, 2012.

"Bravery comes from daring to fail."

—CHRIS BROGAN

CHAPTER 4

Creating Your Digital Footprint

INTRODUCTION

We have selected six social media platforms to guide you in creating your digital footprint. These applications offer a wide range of content creation options. Some, such as LinkedIn, focus on professional networking, while others, YouTube for example, offer limitless opportunities for you to create content for your patients. What all of these sites have in common is the ability for you to write your own story and for your practice to appear high in search engine rankings.

You will notice that one of the most visible aspects of your online presence is not being addressed here—your website. There are several reasons for this. First, a website is static, and thus not by itself a component of social media. Second, creating a viable website can be time- and labor-intensive, requiring Internet knowledge beyond the scope of the typical healthcare provider. The focus of this chapter is on using free online platforms that don't require high-end Web proficiency, yet deliver maximal digital impact for your professional online presence.

If you already have a visible website that ranks well in search engines, congratulations. You're already ahead of the curve. Integrating social media sites with your website will take your online presence up several levels and amplify your digital footprint. So if you choose to create content on the sites profiled here, be sure to link them to your website.

BRANDING STRATEGIES

Using social media is one of the major ways that physicians can brand themselves. Brands used to be mainly about things—mostly consumer products—or corporations. Branding, according to Entrepeneur.com, can be defined as the marketing practice of creating a name, symbol, or design that identifies and differentiates a product from other products.

Think about what brand identity means to you and the purchasing decisions you make. Consider the cars, clothes, food, and beverages that you buy. You might think a brand is mostly about a logo or slogan. It's really much more than that. Leading marketing guru Seth Godin goes further with the idea, by saying that a brand's value can be seen in how often people "choose the expectations, memories, stories and relationships of one brand over the alternatives."[1]

In recent years, the concept has been increasingly applied to people. Doctors brand themselves by their specialty and specific area of expertise—and by reputation. One of the reasons online reputation management is so important is that it can make or break a brand—your medical practice is no exception. Social media can be an effective way to further your brand identity in the market. It gives you an opportunity to position your practice and differentiate yourself from other physicians who practice in your field (aka the competition).

A strong digital presence can also enhance your brand by building patient loyalty, strengthening the relationship you have with current patients, boosting your online presence, and making you more credible in the eyes of patients and peers alike. Identify what's unique about you and your practice. Consider these questions as you build your own brand identity:

- What are your major strengths?
- What does your practice offer that others may not?
- Do you have subspecialty expertise that sets you apart from other practitioners?
- Do you have a hobby or expertise outside of medicine that people might find interesting?
- What are the key messages you want to communicate?

Once you have defined your brand, you can use social media to promote and maintain it. Here, it's important to be consistent in all of your communications, both the content and the design. Choose a template that coordinates with your website and other social media accounts. Develop a tag line for your online persona (for me, it's "social media's leading physician voice").

Branding is not a logo; it's a value proposition.

LINKEDIN: YOUR PROFESSIONAL NETWORK

LinkedIn is one of the simplest and most professional ways for physicians to have a digital footprint. Launched in 2003, long before Facebook and Twitter, it is now the world's largest professional network, with over 175 million members worldwide, and membership is growing every day. LinkedIn reports that professionals are signing up at a rate of approximately two new members per *second*. While many physicians haven't used this tool, it is increasingly a reliable platform for professional networking. The user is in control of the information contained in his or her profile, and in what information is shared as part of a public profile and what is available only for those connected to the user. Remember that LinkedIn is a site for professional networking, so keeping your information private defeats the purpose of joining the service! You can edit any part of your profile at any time. Even if you would just as soon not network, having a profile on LinkedIn lets you make your basic CV information available in an effective way that is not time consuming to maintain.

LinkedIn is essentially an online résumé. Getting started is as simple as listing your current and past positions, along with the dates of employment or affiliation, and including your education, degrees granted, and the years attended. You are under no obligation to include every detail. For example, if you would rather not list the dates you attended medical school, you can just include the names of the institution and degree granted. In addition to the résumé-like listing of your professional experience, you should write a summary paragraph or two.

Unlike other social media sites, you have complete control of how your information appears on LinkedIn. There are no comments or "likes" on individual profiles; those options exist only on the updates you post in your Activity section. (People also have the option to like or comment on anything you post on a group page.) You can write recommendations for others and invite people to recommend you, but you first approve any content before posting.

Experts believe that physicians have been slow to join LinkedIn because it doesn't connect them to patients and is, therefore, not a tool for building one's practice. But there are several reasons why LinkedIn is one of the best sites for healthcare professionals in all fields to use:

1. It is easy to use and navigate.
2. LinkedIn ranks high in Google searches so just having a presence there almost guarantees that your LinkedIn profile will be a page 1 result, ahead of online review sites.
3. Should you ever decide to move or seek another job, LinkedIn can give you a jump start by making relevant connections.
4. If you don't have a website or are part of a large group practice, your LinkedIn page can be a "homepage" just for you. You can link all of your other social media accounts to it and create a personalized link for your page.
5. You're in control!

Essentials

If you are not familiar with LinkedIn, you may want to spend some time exploring the site. You will not be able to see as many profiles or any connections you may already have with colleagues who are already on LinkedIn until you sign up for membership. But you can get some basic guidelines from tutorials on the site before you join. Simply go to http://learn.linkedin.com/profiles/overview and select from among a group of very short (less than one minute each) tutorials on each aspect of a LinkedIn profile. There are other tutorials as well for other features of the site, such as groups, company pages, answers, account settings, and account types. LinkedIn is a free service but it offers a paid premium service that offers more powerful search capabilities, enhanced communication features, and increased access to LinkedIn users. For our LinkedIn essentials guide, we will stick to the free version.

Table 1 shows the number of members and groups in several medical-related categories. The numbers reflect members who used the words listed in the table somewhere in their profiles. You will not be alone on LinkedIn!

Step 1: Sign up. Until you sign up for an account, the information you'll be able to see about other people will be limited. Go to www.linkedin.com. You will be asked for some basic information—your name and e-mail address. You'll then be asked to create a password. That's it—you've now joined LinkedIn!

TABLE 1. Some Healthcare Groups on LinkedIn

Category	No. of Members
Individuals	
Medical	3,428,118
Healthcare	1,445,196
Doctor	687,702
Physician	359,196
Groups	
Medical	11,444
Healthcare	4919
Doctors	1518
Physicians	1436

Source: LinkedIn, July 5, 2012.

Step 2: Spend some time looking at other people's profiles. Start by searching for people you know. You will likely find that you are already connected to many of them, through other people that you know in common. As you scroll through the profiles of people you know, a box will appear on the side to tell you how you are connected to that person. Note also the variances in profiles. Some people include detailed summaries, honors and awards, organizations of which they are members, key word lists of skills, and recommendations they have written for others or recommendations written by others for them. Don't be too daunted by this complexity—it simply shows you the range of options you'll have in developing a profile that suits you and the possibilities offered by the LinkedIn service (see examples in Figures 4.1A and 4.1B).

Step 3: Gather your information. This step should be relatively easy. You already know most of it; grab a copy of your résumé or CV, and you will have most of what you need. However, there is one key piece of your LinkedIn profile that you should spend some time thinking about before you write it, and that's the summary. As you build your profile, LinkedIn will prompt you to write your summary by asking you to summarize yourself and your objectives.

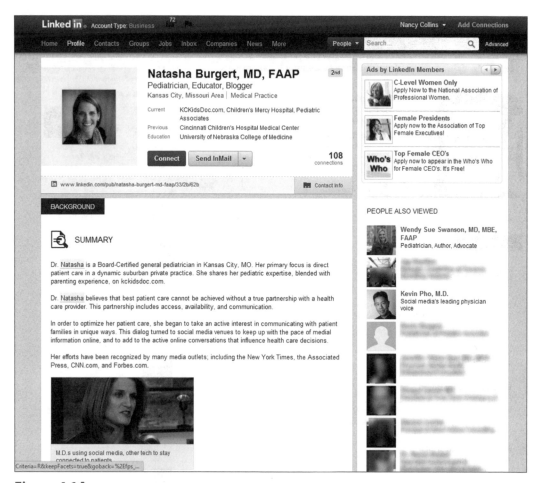

Figure 4.1A

Don't be tempted to gloss over this aspect of your profile; it can actually be the most important part! You can break up the text with headings to focus the reader's attention on the aspects of your career or practice that you most want to highlight. Often, a summary is only 100 to 200 words, but it can be longer if you prefer. Be sure to include key words in the summary. See how other healthcare professionals (especially those in the same field) have crafted their summaries. Here is where you can tell an interesting story about yourself, highlight some unique element of your practice, or mention blogs you write for. You can put your personal stamp on the summary in ways that aren't possible with the rest of the profile, which uses a more traditional résumé-like format. So spend some time making it a powerful statement.

Step 4: Complete your profile. LinkedIn will first ask for your e-mail address and password and give you an opportunity to immediately start adding contacts from your address book. However, you can skip this step until you've completed your profile. For building your profile, you will be asked for information about your experience, education, and skills and to post a photo. You can also add information on:

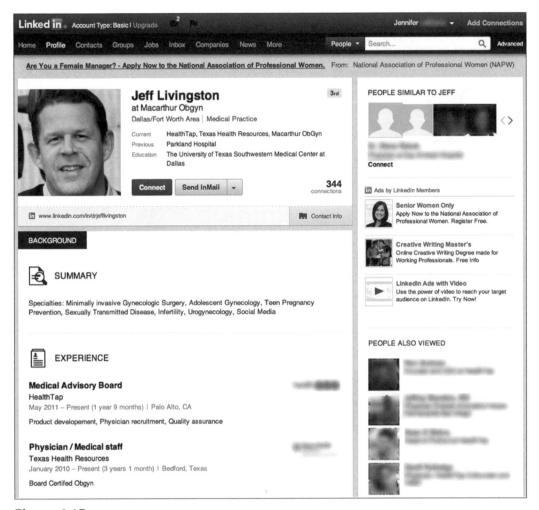

Figure 4.1B

- Projects;
- Languages spoken;
- Publications;
- Organizations;
- Honors and awards;
- Certifications; and
- Volunteer positions and causes.

LinkedIn's program takes you through the various sections of the profile and tells you what you've completed and what is still left to do as you make your way through. You can stop at any time and complete the profile in stages. However, if you do that, we recommend that you not allow your profile to be posted on the site until you have completed it. An incomplete profile will not enhance your reputation and could send the wrong message to people who come across it when doing a search for you.

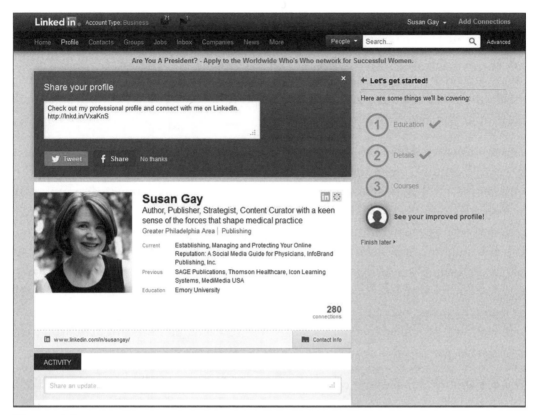

Figure 4.2

You can see the completeness of your profile on the right side of the "Edit Profile" page. If you have to write your profile in stages, picking up where you left off is easy. The program will automatically take you back to incomplete sections. Once each major section is complete, a check will appear next to it, as shown in Figure 4.2. You can also choose how you want the public to see your profile. You can limit access to your connections, for example.

LinkedIn helps you build your profile by providing you with a measure called Profile Strength. The meter on the right side of your profile will let you know how robust your profile is. As you add more content, your profile strength increases. By placing your cursor over the circle in the box, you can view the next level of strength you can reach. LinkedIn also provides a link to "Improve Your Profile Strength" for more information to guide you through adding more content to your profile.

Step 5: Get connections. Once you are satisfied with your profile, it's time to get connections. This is cyberspace, where connections are made with the click of a mouse. In fact, LinkedIn's algorithms will help you build your list of connections with relative ease by suggesting colleagues, fellow alumni, and others who share some aspect of your history. You can import your address list as a starting point to see all the people you know who are already on LinkedIn and then select those you wish to invite to join your trusted network. You can also search for classmates from college and medical school or search for people by name, the same as you may have done when you were looking for sample profiles. Soon, though, LinkedIn will have hundreds of additional suggestions, culled from your connections' network and listed as "People You May Know."

Connections are labeled as "1st degree," meaning they are a direct connection to you; "2nd degree," meaning they are linked to one of your direct connections; or "3rd degree," which means that someone in your network is connected to someone in their network. It's likely that you have never heard of most of your third-degree connections. As a general rule, it is best to invite connections only from people you know through work or school or have met at a meeting. Although you are likely to get lots of invitations from strangers wanting to join your network, you should not seek to connect with people you do not know. The exception to this guideline would be if you are trying to connect with the proverbial "friend of a friend," in which case you may want to add a personal message to the automated LinkedIn invitation that goes to that person when you chose "connect."

You can choose to make your connection list public or you can limit who can see your connections. If you elect to use the privacy feature, only your first-degree connections will be able to see who else you are connected to. In addition, you must approve all connection requests, and you can at any time remove a connection.

LinkedIn will send you a weekly summary including news it thinks might interest you, group updates, and a notification of any changes your connections have made in their profiles. This summary can be scanned quickly and is an efficient way to keep tabs on the people you're connected to.

Maximizing LinkedIn

The steps above will give you a solid profile on LinkedIn and help to establish your online identity, even if you do not use the many other features of the site.

Maintain your profile to make sure it is up to date. Periodically adding information or otherwise updating your profile keeps it active in the search engines and will result in higher placement on search result pages. It also sends a message to both your current connections and anyone who searches for you that you are active in your field and part of a larger community.

Share news and updates. You can share information from anywhere on the Web on LinkedIn. The site offers users a sharing bookmark that you can add to your browser toolbar. Clicking on that tab will bring up a window where you can add a comment

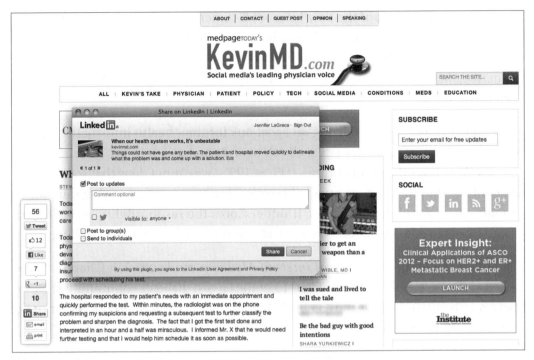

Figure 4.3

and post to your LinkedIn updates, post to a group, or send to an individual. Figure 4.3 shows how this would appear on screen. You can also post updates to Twitter from your LinkedIn status updates, as long as they are within Twitter's 140-character limit.

Join groups. See Table 1 for a list of the number of groups that exist on LinkedIn in various medically related categories. Joining groups of alumni, fellow employees, or groups organized around common interests is a good way to expand your reach and connect with like-minded people. Group pages allow members to share information and comment on it, ask questions, and discuss issues of mutual interest. Some groups are "open," meaning anyone can join; others require approval of the group's manager. Clicking on the group name in a search on LinkedIn's site will either give you immediate access or automatically send a message to the manager for approval of your membership.

FACEBOOK: CONNECT AND SHARE

Facebook is the world's largest social networking website, with over a billion users.[2] Recently, a survey released by the National Research Corporation involving 23,000 patients found that 41% of them use social media sites to look for health information. Of those, nearly 94% said Facebook was their site of choice. It makes intuitive sense, since Facebook is accumulating users at a record pace.[3]

However, Susannah Fox of the Pew Internet & American Life Project doesn't agree with that statistic. I often cite Pew's numbers when doing my social media talks, so I pay attention to what Fox says. According to Pew, in 2009, 39% of patients who went online used social media sites.[4] Of those, only 12% had gotten health information from those sites.

So are patients increasingly relying on Facebook for their health information, as the recent headlines suggest? Or is Facebook over-hyped as a tool for Internet-savvy patients? Whatever the numbers are—94% or 12%—we cannot deny that social media will continue to grow and eventually become a source where a growing number of patients can research health topics. It underscores the responsibility of healthcare professionals to educate patients to critically question what they read online.

Remember the *Journal of General Internal Medicine* study cited in Chapter 1 that looked at the Facebook wall posts from 15 of the largest diabetes communities? More than a quarter of the posts featured non-FDA-approved, "natural" products that could be harmful to diabetic patients.[5]

Also consider that fewer than half of patients always checked the source of the health information they read online.[6] That's unacceptable. As physicians, we need to continue our efforts to get online, get social, and help patients find reputable health data that can potentially affect their health decisions.

Facebook is not just for individuals. Many companies now have a presence on the site, as do federal health agencies and professional associations. The American Medical Association is on Facebook (www.facebook.com/AmericanMedicalAssociation). So is the Centers for Disease Control and Prevention (CDC) (www.facebook.com/CDC). The American Heart Association (AHA) has over 250,000 likes on its Facebook page (www.facebook.com/AmericanHeart). Facebook is ubiquitous and free, and it's relatively easy to set up a page.

Unfortunately, Facebook has also been a minefield of sorts for the medical profession, with infractions ranging from unprofessional conduct by medical students to patient privacy violations by attending physicians.[7] One solution would be for individual doctors to simply avoid Facebook altogether for personal use. That seems a bit drastic. There's no reason why doctors can't participate in the social benefits that Facebook has to offer.

Here's another solution. I embrace the "dual-citizenship" approach, discussed in a 2011 *Annals of Internal Medicine* perspective piece.[8] With Facebook in particular, I recommend that you limit your personal profile to friends and family. These are people who can follow your personal, day-to-day happenings, pictures, and video.

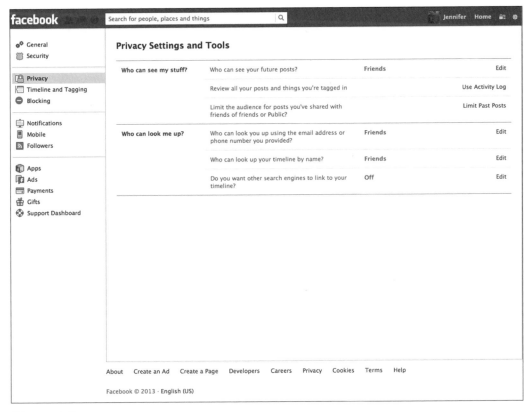

Figure 4.4

Patients should not have access to this personal profile. See Figure 4.4 for options in privacy settings.

After you have secured the privacy of your personal Facebook profile, set up a separate Facebook page for your practice that serves as your public persona. This site will be the one that patients can view. This page needs to be HIPAA-compliant and professionally self-aware. This page can contain information about your practice, feature commentary on news events you care to write about, and be "liked" by anyone without the sharing of personal information. And finally, it's a good idea to check your privacy settings once a week to guard against any changes that may have been inadvertently made to them.

Essentials

The following steps in setting up a professional presence on Facebook are limited to Facebook's pages system, which allows users to create their own "homepage." Pages are used by a wide variety of businesses, organizations, and celebrities; even the President of the United States has this type of Facebook presence. Pages offer several advantages for physicians. As mentioned previously, they allow you to keep your personal and your professional profiles completely separate. There is no limit

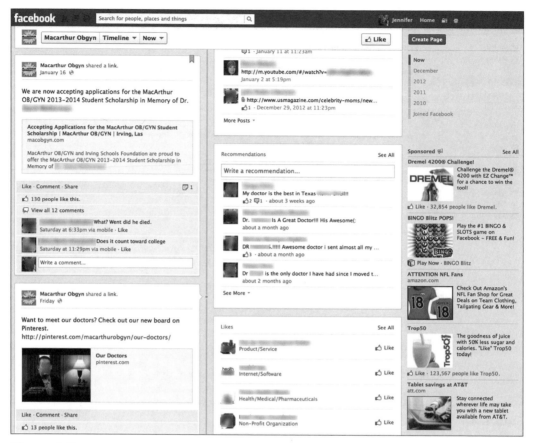

Figure 4.5

to the number of people who can "Like" your page. In fact, that's all people can do. They can't "Friend" you," only "Like" you. The page can be set up to automatically accept new likes so you don't have to accept each request individually, and anyone can view your page at any time. With these steps in mind, you can enjoy the social interaction Facebook has to offer and stay out of professional danger.

Step 1. Look at profiles of physicians in your field. If you are not familiar with Facebook pages, you might want to visit some existing pages before creating your own. In order to craft your own page well, you should visit pages maintained by physicians in your field. Try to find established pages that will have more likes and active participation by visitors. (See Figure 4.5 as an example.) A well-known colleague might have a few thousand likes on his or her page.

The owner of a Facebook page can add information about himself or herself such as birthday, location, and a short bio. A picture to represent the page can also be uploaded. Facebook's "Timeline" system allows owners to attach a large "cover photo" at the top of their page, like the one shown in Figure 4.6, to attract attention from people viewing the page.

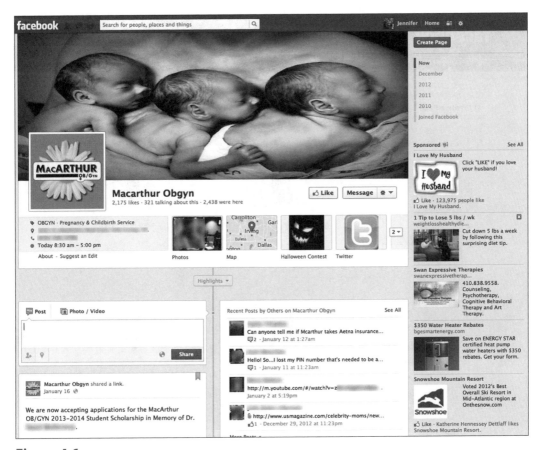

Figure 4.6

Step 2. Select a page type to start creating your page. Go to www.facebook.com/pages/create.php. On this Web page, you can choose the category under which your page will be located. The six categories listed are for local businesses, companies/organizations/institutions, brands or products, public figures, entertainment, and causes or communities. The most likely choice for you will be local business. Then select the appropriate category from the drop-down menu. Each category comes loaded with tools to help you create your page. You must supply basic information of practice name, address, and phone number before you can proceed (see Figure 4.7). But you can skip over the prompts for adding a profile picture and filling in the About section for now. When you set up a business page, Facebook automatically includes tools that will help you provide information to your followers, such as hours of operation and services offered, in a clear and easy-to-find way.

These tools will also make it easier for you to showcase any promotions you are running, patient success stories, impressive before and after pictures (with patient permission!), or related material such as new advances in your field.

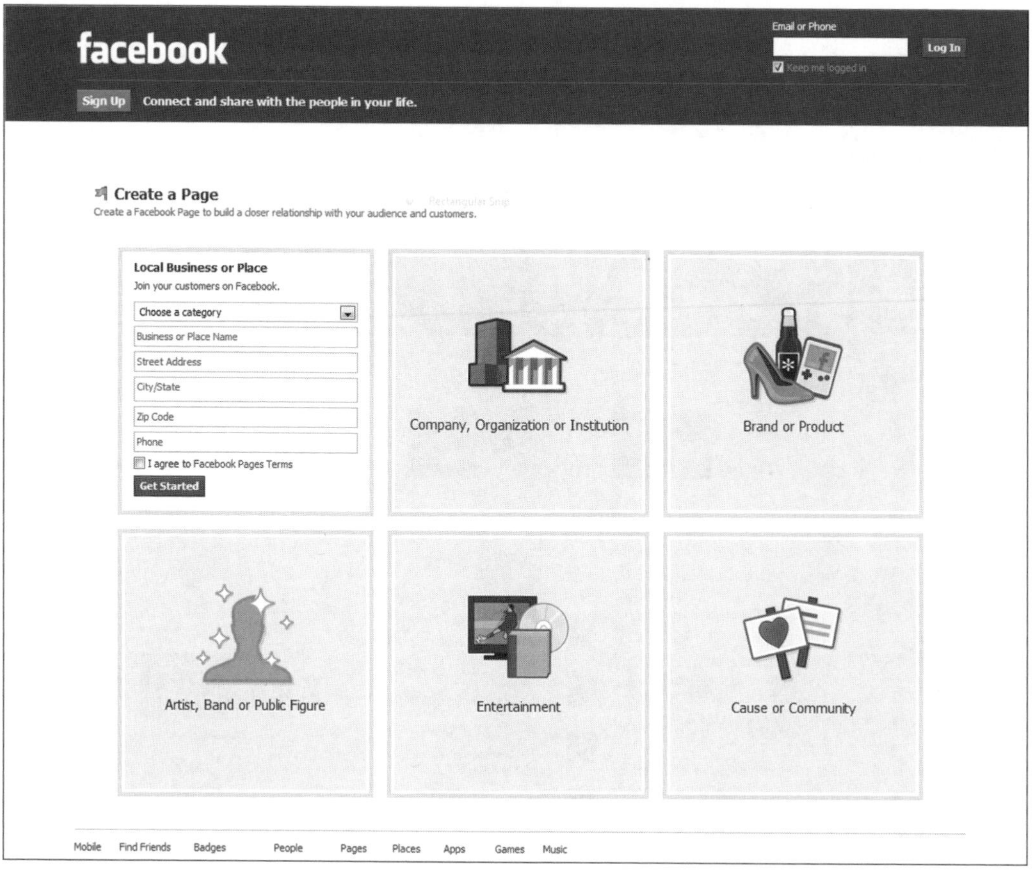

Figure 4.7

Step 3. Add information about you and your practice. This information is not required for your page to be operational. However, it is highly recommended, especially the About section. This is a basic summary of yourself and your work, much like the Summary section of a LinkedIn profile. You can even use the same description as you use on LinkedIn. Some experts believe that consistency of information across your social network is not only a good way to build brand identity but increases the chances of being highly ranked by search engines. Adding photos is a must. See Figure 4.8 for the About section of my Facebook page.

Maximizing Facebook

Make connections with other social media. You can add a Like button that links your Facebook page to your website by going to "Promote this page on your web site" under "Getting Started" on Facebook. Go to "Core Concepts," then "Social Plugins." Follow the instructions to add a "Like Box" to your website. You can also connect your Facebook page to your Twitter page or add your Facebook address to your LinkedIn page.

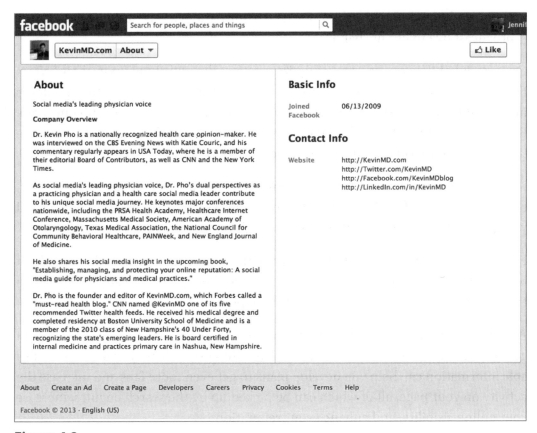

facebook   Search for people, places and things   Q   Jennif

KevinMD.com   About ▾   👍 Like

About

Social media's leading physician voice

Company Overview

Dr. Kevin Pho is a nationally recognized health care opinion-maker. He was interviewed on the CBS Evening News with Katie Couric, and his commentary regularly appears in USA Today, where he is a member of their editorial Board of Contributors, as well as CNN and the New York Times.

As social media's leading physician voice, Dr. Pho's dual perspectives as a practicing physician and a health care social media leader contribute to his unique social media journey. He keynotes major conferences nationwide, including the PRSA Health Academy, Healthcare Internet Conference, Massachusetts Medical Society, American Academy of Otolaryngology, Texas Medical Association, the National Council for Community Behavioral Healthcare, PAINWeek, and New England Journal of Medicine.

He also shares his social media insight in the upcoming book, "Establishing, managing, and protecting your online reputation: A social media guide for physicians and medical practices."

Dr. Pho is the founder and editor of KevinMD.com, which Forbes called a "must-read health blog." CNN named @KevinMD one of its five recommended Twitter health feeds. He received his medical degree and completed residency at Boston University School of Medicine and is a member of the 2010 class of New Hampshire's 40 Under Forty, recognizing the state's emerging leaders. He is board certified in internal medicine and practices primary care in Nashua, New Hampshire.

Basic Info

Joined Facebook   06/13/2009

Contact Info

Website   http://KevinMD.com
http://Twitter.com/KevinMD
http://Facebook.com/KevinMDblog
http://LinkedIn.com/in/KevinMD

About   Create an Ad   Create a Page   Developers   Careers   Privacy   Cookies   Terms   Help

Facebook © 2013 · English (US)

Figure 4.8

Share news and exclusive content. Starting "Discussions" on your page can be a good way to involve viewers of your page. Try to select topics that are both relevant and engaging to increase participation. Here are some recent examples of the types of Facebook posts on some medical practice pages and the comments they generated:

- *Boon for Bloomberg: Studies Show Soda Contributes to Child Obesity:* Post on Pediatric Associates Kansas City's Facebook page with a link to a *Time* magazine article. This post generated six comments, including parents asking about alternatives such as juices. The practice physicians then responded with a link to American Academy of Pediatrics' recommendations for juice.[9]

- *Flu Shots and Football? It Must Be Fall!:* Post on Pediatric Associates Kansas City's Facebook page with a link to its blog post on this topic.[9]

- *How Often Do You Need to See Me?:* Post on the Facebook page of urologist Neil Baum, MD, with a link to his blog post on this topic.[10]

- *A Great Military Delivery Story in Honor of Memorial Day. We Love and Support Our Troops:* Facebook post on MacArthur OB/GYN's Facebook page with a link to blog post entitled "Technology Brings Dad into Delivery Room via Skype Linking

Irving and South Korea," about a MacArthur patient's recent delivery that was broadcast live to her husband.[11]

Once people Like you, any status updates you make will show up in their "News Feed," which runs down the center of their page. Making regular status updates is important for maintaining a presence and reminding people you are still out there. Best practices suggest you should post something every other day if you have the time, but no less than once a week in order to stay visible.

Keep your posts professional. Let your patients know about new services you offer, or comment on medical findings in the news. Always be sure to portray yourself and your practice in a professional and positive light.

For practices that may be hesitant to let patients comment on their wall or that don't have the resources to fully engage patients on Facebook, settings can be adjusted so that only the page administrator is allowed to post content.

Analyze key metrics. Facebook offers tools to help you analyze key metrics. You can get insights into who visits your page and what they do while they're on it. This valuable information can help you develop plans to get even more fans and increase the activity on your page, all of which can be picked up by the search engines, increase your online visibility, and enhance your reputation.

Jeff Livingston, MD, of MacArthur OB/GYN talks about how Facebook plays a vital role in his professional social media strategy:

> **Patients have moved beyond simply reading about health information on the Web. They now want an interactive experience. Embrace this excitement. Own your online reputation by providing the online information your patients are asking for. Your patients should not have to rely on Wikipedia to know what to do. They should be able to get high-quality information directly from you. By getting involved in social media, you can promote your area of expertise and define your image. You can create your own digital footprint. You can improve patient education, increase referrals, promote practice loyalty, and increase utilization of services leading to practice growth.**
>
> **This has worked well for MacArthur OB/GYN. By providing high-quality health information on our website, podcasts, and social media channels and by the innovative use of technology in the office, we are helping our patients make better-informed decisions.**

For the most part, I manage content by myself. But over the years, the other doctors have gotten administration privileges on our Facebook page to also help manage content. The doctors, nurse practitioner, and midwife all blog, which has been very helpful. I think it is important to have providers manage the content so that the voice stays authentic. I think this also helps a practice stay focused on the idea of patient engagement and patient education without crossing over the line and focusing on practice marketing.

I think it is important for providers to make social media a part of their daily routine—a way of life—so it does not become a job or just another thing you have to do. I check our Facebook page daily on my iPhone. I keep Tweetdeck open on my desktop. If something pops into my head or I feel inspired then I post. If not, then I go about my daily routine. This makes updating our social media presence fun and not a chore. Finding great tools like Tumblr, Tweetdeck, and the Facebook pages app is key to being able to update multiple sources in one click. This minimizes the amount of time required. I spend less than one hour a day unless I am writing a blog post.

I love the interaction and community aspect of social media. I don't like to just push out information, although I do think this has tremendous value for patient education and to improve the quality of online medical information. I really enjoy when you get a push-pull. Doctors can learn from patients just as much as patients can learn from us. The other day I was at home thinking about miscarriages and how we talk to patients. I posted about it on our Facebook page. It was amazing to hear women talking about what doctors said that helped and what doctors said that made things worse. This is social media working the way it is supposed to.

The effect of social media on our practice is beyond belief. We have doubled our office size three times in the past six years. We have gone from a group of three doctors to a group of seven doctors, one nurse practitioner, and one certified nurse manager, and we are still growing.

Jeff Livingston, MD
Obstetrician-Gynecologist
Irving, Texas
http://macobgyn.com
www.facebook.com/macobgyn

YOUTUBE: BROADCAST YOUR PRACTICE

YouTube is the Internet's leading video streaming service. Millions of videos are hosted on YouTube, with more being added every day; these videos can range from having tens to hundreds of millions of views. Furthermore, YouTube is the number 2 search engine on the Web.[12] More than 800 million users watch more than four billion hours of video each month on YouTube. Traffic from mobile devices tripled in 2011. It is the third most visited website in both the United States and worldwide.[13]

Before you decide to skip this section because you have no intention of making videos of yourself, note the following:

- You do not need to make your own videos to have a presence on YouTube! But, ultimately, your online presence will be enhanced if you do.
- You do not have to personally appear in any video you do make.

In other words, you have many options of how to interact with this key social media outlet, and you can increase your presence incrementally once you are more comfortable with it. YouTube can be a useful tool for physicians, because video is an important means for representing your practice on the Internet. Videos help patients make a personal connection to your practice. YouTube is also a good place to post updated medical stories and key information, such as vaccine updates or cancer screening guidelines. The impact of loading videos on YouTube can be seen in these statistics: 100 million people take some action on YouTube every week, such as sharing, liking, or adding comments. More than 50% of videos on YouTube have been rated or include comments from the community.[13]

A recent study by AMN Healthcare, a staffing agency, found that physicians and other healthcare professionals are also using YouTube to make professional connections—without actually making a video themselves. In a survey of nearly 2800 healthcare professionals, the study showed that 29% are using YouTube in this manner. It's interesting to note that just 23% said they use LinkedIn for connecting with colleagues.[14] This finding doesn't mean that nearly one-third of healthcare professionals are actually posting videos. Physicians who make videos are in the minority, but those who do can become established as experts in their field, making it possible for other practitioners to find them, comment on videos, add perspective, and share the videos with patients and other colleagues. Videos, including posting *and* sharing, increase your chances of being found in a search.

Don't think that the majority of YouTube videos are lighthearted or inconsequential. Universities post academic lectures from professors, and many hospitals post videos for patients to show the facilities and provide details of the services they offer. The AHA chose YouTube as its medium to push chest-only CPR. Instead of doing a television spot or a radio commercial, or placing a newspaper ad, the AHA created a YouTube video featuring Ken Jeong, a comedian, actor, *and* family physician. In the span of a few weeks, the video had over 400,000 views! YouTube is part of the social media network that allows doctors to carry their messages directly to patients.

Consider this scenario: A patient comes to you for a specific surgical procedure, but does not know anything about the procedure and is understandably a little apprehensive. Imagine pulling out your tablet or laptop and showing this patient a video of that procedure. Do you think interacting this way with your patient in the exam room before the surgery will build trust and improve patient satisfaction?

Well, yes it does. A study from the *Journal of the American College of Surgeons* found that patients who watched a preparation video before their operation reported less anxiety about the procedure and higher rates of satisfaction with the surgical experience. They even reported less pain after the operation.[15]

YouTube is catalogued by the search engines; relevant videos will be prominently displayed—most likely on the first page—of search engine results. The results might be shown as a thumbnail of a video that meets the criteria for a keyword search. Because many practices are not yet incorporating videos into their Internet strategy, you will have a good chance of being highlighted in the search results if you use YouTube.

Video is not difficult or expensive to do. While there is a place for both professionally created and self-recorded video, the guidelines on YouTube are intended to help you get the best results without having to make an enormous investment in equipment or professional services.

Social media experts suggest building your personal brand by creating your own videos to show your expertise, make potential patients feel more connected to you, and build your practice. Only you can decide if this social media outlet fits you and your practice's goals. The following guidelines offer suggestions on getting on YouTube, creating a channel, and building that channel with your own content.

Essentials

Step 1. Create an account. At www.youtube.com, you can sign in with your Google login information if you already have a Google account because YouTube is owned by Google. If you do not have a Google account, when prompted to sign in, you can click there and go to "Create Account" at the top-right of the page.

The Google username you create when signing up does not have to be your public name on YouTube. You can choose a different YouTube username when you create your channel (see below). Once you submit all the required information and agree to follow the terms, Google will offer you a text or voice call option to verify your new account. Once verified, you can move to the next step of setting up a profile.

Step 2. Create a profile. You are given the opportunity here to create a profile. Or use the one you may already have for Google+. You can skip this step for now if you wish and create a profile when you customize your channel (more on that below).

Step 3. Browse videos. Before you begin thinking about the types of video you could upload to YouTube, you should spend some time looking at current offerings on the site. If you have not viewed many YouTube videos or have not done so recently, start by searching for some videos in your area of expertise. You can type a name, subject, keyword, or video title into the search box at the top of YouTube's homepage. You can then narrow your results by using the filter function that allows you to sort or explore related content areas. For example, if you are a pediatrician wanting to see videos on YouTube relevant to that patient group, you can see what's been posted recently and which videos are rated highest. You can also focus on specific aspects of the field such as fine motor skills or the neurologic examination.

Step 4. Customize your channel. Click on your username at the top of the screen to be taken to your YouTube account. Under the YouTube heading, on the right, click "My Channel." Your channel was automatically created when you created your account.

Your channel is your home for broadcasting on YouTube. It's the place to house the videos you make ("Uploads"), the videos you love ("Favorites"), and the videos you've organized ("Playlists"). Personalize your channel by selecting the background color, formatting, and module options. You can preview the settings you've selected and see how you'll appear on YouTube. If you haven't yet uploaded a photo or completed a profile, you will have the option to do that before moving on.

Your channel is likely also the landing page that people will find if they search for you on YouTube. In creating your channel, think carefully about how you want to position yourself. This is where you (or your practice) become a brand. If you already have a brand established through your website, you can carry that identity over to your YouTube channel by being consistent with your choices of colors and designs.

You do not need to fill in much information on your YouTube channel. There is space for a short bio, plus areas to fill in your city and country if desired. Click on the "Edit" button next to your name to complete a brief profile, so that viewers can distinguish you and your channel from the millions of other videos vying for their attention. Next, go to "Channel Settings" in the upper left, where you will find three tabs for customizing your channel:

- **Appearance.** In the Appearance tab of the Channel Settings view, you can choose a background image and a color scheme for your channel. Any time you are setting up appearance features, it's a good idea to make them consistent with the images and graphics associated with your practice. This will strengthen you brand identity.
- **Information and settings.** Be sure to give your channel a name and description that make sense. This information will appear wherever your channel is found on YouTube and is also displayed in the "About" section on your channel. The title you choose will be shown at the top of your channel, next to your avatar, so make it good! The channel name can be your name or another name, but make sure it is descriptive. The character count of the channel description is 1000 characters, but only 250 characters will be exposed by default in the About section, with the remainder available behind a "more" link. Be sure to write a concise and useful description; this shortened version of the description will also appear across the site. In this section, you can update or enhance your profile. A link takes you back to the Google profile page. You can add more information on your practice and education. You can also add personal details if you wish, but keep in mind that you will be hosting a professional channel for your practice. You can also create a custom URL here. Once created, the URL for that specific channel cannot be changed. Give your channel descriptive tags that allow it to show up to users doing a search. As with specific video tags, when users type keywords related to your video, your channel can appear in their search results.
- **Tabs.** Here you can decide if you would like to showcase a Featured tab. Clicking into the Featured tab lets you choose the template that best displays your content. YouTube now has three templates you can choose from: Overview, Blogger, and Everything. Every template in the Featured tab has a featured video player so you can give your users a glimpse of what kind of content is in your channel. Each template displays content differently and showcases certain types of content more prominently than others. You should take into consideration the amount and type of content you have when making a template decision.

When you are finished customizing your channel, be sure to click "Done Editing" on the far right to save your changes. Figure 4.9 shows an example of a YouTube channel created by a physician.

Step 5. Make videos! Now that you have seen numerous videos, you may be thinking that you should be delivering your own message to your patients. You've probably seen some poor-quality videos and concluded that you can do better. The videos you make can answer questions, provide basic information, or just present a short update. The content needs to be interesting and compelling, or entertaining if appropriate for the subject matter. (The box Tips for Effective YouTube Content on page 78 has some tips on creating good material for YouTube videos.)

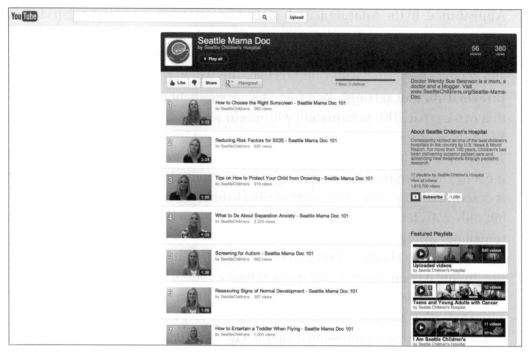

Figure 4.9

TIPS FOR EFFECTIVE YOUTUBE CONTENT

1. Make it relevant. Be sure to stick to issues that you know patients are concerned about or that are instructive about your practice.
2. Don't use YouTube videos to replace important text but to enhance it. Some people learn best watching a video; others don't. So if you are communicating important information about your practice or want patients to take some action as a result of seeing the video, be sure to include this information as text content somewhere on your website or your practice's Facebook page.
3. Be mindful of length. If the video is an academic lecture or even a talk to a consumer group, you can include the entire talk. But if the content is tips for patients on flu shots, it's best to keep the video to fewer than three minutes.
4. Tags should be clear and concise. Remember, people will likely find your videos through a keyword search, so make sure you have used tags that are simply and explicitly related to the content. Use a title that is clear and concise.
5. Use your editing software to add your practice's logo or other brand identity during the opening and closing credits or on every screen.

VIDEO TIPS

1. Beware of any background noise. Examples include air conditioners, loud computer humming, road noise, and walking noises. Close doors if possible to avoid excess noise.
2. Avoid stripes and other detailed patterns on clothes. Complicated backgrounds are difficult to reproduce on cameras that have fewer pixels per inch.
3. Make a teleprompter. If you've created a script in advance, you can make it a PowerPoint file and use it as a teleprompter (out of sight, of course) during filming.
4. Talk slowly and speak clearly. People often talk faster on camera. If you are a fast talker anyway, practice speaking more slowly. Thirty seconds of video should contain 65 to 78 words; 60 seconds should have 130 to 155 words.[17]

Video equipment should not be a major obstacle, although most experts advise against using a webcam to create videos. A simple video camera will produce high-quality video. Many portable video cameras now record in high definition. Even smartphones, such as the iPhone and many Android-based phones, record in HD. Try these options first. If you want to produce truly professional videos, you will need to either invest in equipment, including lighting and sound, or hire a professional videographer. Of course, the advantage to making your own videos is that you can delete and start over as many times as you want without incurring costs until you get a final version worth posting. You can also make and post new videos at any time of the day or night to provide context to medical news stories or post timely practice updates. See Video Tips above for more helpful advice.

Most computers come with software to help you edit a self-made video. You can even add a title frame, text subtitle, and images to your clip. Once your video is edited, you are ready to upload to YouTube.

If you do not want to be seen or heard, you can still make videos. Free software, such as Screencast-O-Matic (www.screencast-o-matic.com), allows you to record webcasts of PowerPoint presentations or anything else you create on your computer. This alternative means you can create video content for your website without personally appearing onscreen.

Neil Baum, MD, is a urologist at Touro Infirmary in New Orleans, Louisiana, and author of *Marketing Your Clinical Practice: Ethically, Effectively, Economically*, 4th Edition. He recently offered some practical tips for creating patient education videos on YouTube[16]:

Videos are an excellent method of attracting new patients and educating existing ones. Creating a script is the first step. By following a few guidelines, you can create a compelling video that will result in improvement in educating the public and the patients in your practice.

Start by defining the condition. For example, "Hematuria is the condition where there is blood in the urine, and the urine turns red or dark brown. This is not a normal situation and requires an evaluation to find the cause of the problem."

Now write a few sentences about the condition itself, including other lay terms for the medical condition, and describe the anatomy involved or even link the term to a news story or something patients are familiar with from popular culture. If you are discussing testicular tumors you might mention that Dan Abrams had testicular cancer and is cured of his disease.

Next provide the signs and symptoms of the condition. (For example, "What are the signs and symptoms of kidney stones?") Describe what the patient will feel or see. Is there pain with the condition? Does the patient feel something abnormal or just see something abnormal? Are there some misconceptions about the symptoms that should be cleared up? Are any particular symptoms more ominous than others? Are there other conditions that might be confused with the condition?

Now tell the viewer how the condition is diagnosed. For this segment, describe how doctors diagnose this problem. What are the typical history and physical exam findings? More importantly, what can a patient expect— imaging, blood work, diagnostic biopsy, or other invasive procedures? Are the tests done on site or is another appointment required? How long will patients have to wait for results?

Finally describe how the condition is treated. Describe both conservative and aggressive treatment options. What are the pros and cons of each method of treatment? Describe the typical or likely outcome in most cases. Describe what patients can expect during a procedure and during the course of treatment, and what the total recovery time will be. You should also mention the risks and complications of the various treatment options. You will also want to mention in this segment any alternative types of treatment and what will happen if patients ignore your advice or don't get treated.

It is very effective if you can include a patient providing a testimonial about what it was like before, during, and after treatment.

I suggest ending each video with a call to action. For example, my videos end with, "I know you may have some additional questions regarding <name the condition>, and I suggest you go to my website, or you are welcome to call my office to make an appointment so that we might discuss <name the condition> further. I look forward to meeting with you."

Time yourself, as these videos should be 7 to 10 minutes in length. Any longer, you will lose your viewer, and he or she will either click off of your video or start thinking about something else.

Neil Baum, MD
Urologist
New Orleans, Louisiana
www.neilbaum.com

Maximizing YouTube

Post videos often. To make the most of your YouTube channel, post as many videos as you can. Your directory of videos can be a helpful resource for patients and colleagues searching your channel. Uploading monthly or weekly update or tip videos is a great idea; timeliness can keep you on the first page of search results.

Share videos. To get the most out of your YouTube videos, you need to promote your channel so that people can find you. YouTube has features that help you get started in the promotion process. Sharing on other social media sites where you already have a presence is a good place to start. You can share your videos immediately after you create and post them by going into your YouTube account settings and selecting "Sharing." Using this menu, you can automatically share you videos through Facebook, Twitter, and Google Reader. Consider your audience before sharing, though. Don't post a video to your personal Facebook account, but to your professional Facebook page where your patients can see it when they search for you or your practice.

You can also share your videos on a blog by going to your YouTube account settings and selecting "Blog Setup." This option allows you to link your YouTube to your blog and post videos on your blog. You can embed videos on a blog or on your website.

Once you have established how you want to share your YouTube videos, you can further promote them by creating more links. The more links you have to each video, the higher it will rank with search engines. Opportunities for linking include your

LinkedIn profile, your e-mail signature, and any presentations you give. Commenting on related videos and leaving a link to your video is also a way to promote your videos.

Let's look at how two physicians have successfully incorporated YouTube into their practice:

I started a YouTube channel in February 2011. Just like the blog that I have, the YouTube channel is a simple, grassroots effort. I make the video myself using a Flip cam, my husband does brief edits with iMovie, and it's published. The content often complements my blog posts on topics I think are better shared visually. I have no "staff," and do not discuss content with any outside parties. Both my blog and the YouTube videos are simply reflections of what I want to share.

I love the opportunity to share relevant medical information in a succinct and shareable format. It is very easy for me to share the information on my WordPress blog or on our practice's Facebook page/Twitter account. In addition, I have the URL available to my patients as they arrive at the office so they can watch the video on their smartphone while they wait; this is a huge time saver for me.

My blog and YouTube videos are some of the first things new patients mention upon arriving at the clinic. In my opinion, if patients come to see me because of a video they have seen, that's great. However, my goal for my online work is not to market myself or attract new families. My goal is to spread and share important, evidenced-based healthcare information to my community. Period. And if a new patient thinks that's cool, we will get along just fine!

I update the YouTube channel every six to eight weeks. Each video takes roughly two hours for me to put together (content, filming, and editing). My only regret is not having enough time to be able to do more videos.

Natasha Burgert, MD
Pediatrician
Kansas City, Missouri
http://kckidsdoc.com
www.youtube.com/user/KCKidsDoc?feature=watch

In 2011, I started the Mama Doc 101 series, about 18 months after starting the Mama Doc blog. However, before starting the series, I had created a number of videos that I'd filmed spontaneously in response to new information (suffocations in slings), topics I thought needed more exposure (preparing for disasters), or hot topics (like my take against chocolate toddler "formula" being marketed to parents).

The reason I started the Mama Doc 101 series was to capture some of the things I say over and over again in the office and collect them in one place. Ultimately, I wanted to tell it like it is, just like I do in clinic, online.

I do all the videos on my own without a script. Sometimes I do two to three takes, but usually I do only one. I want the video to be authentic and real, not scripted with a canned marketing style like so much advice we find online. In the beginning, I did a lot of the filming with a Flip camera and would even edit the video on my own. However, now I have an assistant who runs the camera, puts titles at the beginning and end of the videos, and uploads the videos to YouTube.

I film a video about once a week. I usually film them in bundles. (Sometimes I change clothes to mask that.) I usually film three videos in about 30 to 45 minutes. But I will prep for the videos in advance, sometimes spending two to three hours reading studies, policy statements, and websites.

I find it valuable to send my patients to the links. Unfortunately, with an electronic medical records system in the exam room that blocks social media and YouTube in particular, I can't show the videos in clinic. Usually I have patients find them on Google. In their after-visit summary, I'll type "Google 'Protecting Infants From The Sun, Seattle Mama Doc'" so they can easily find the video. It's not perfect, but it's better than nothing. I often explain the same things in the office, but I love the repository of content out there that can support their learning at home or with their spouse/partner who is also raising the child.

My practice has been packed full since I started the Mama Doc series, so much so that I don't currently accept new patients. The business case for social media is that it allows you to stand out, provide more personal and comprehensive care, and ultimately partner with patients in a unique way.

Wendy Sue Swanson, MD
Pediatrician
Seattle, Washington
http://seattlemamadoc.seattlechildrens.org
www.youtube.com/playlist?list=PLFDF0A4E130F59AEF&feature=plcp

TWITTER: WHAT'S HAPPENING NOW

Twitter is a social media service that allows users to communicate with one another by composing tweets, short messages of up to 140 characters. Despite that limitation, tweets can convey important information and often include links, video, and photos. Twitter has captured the mainstream imagination, with celebrities and news organizations embracing the medium. It is one of today's most popular social media websites and claims almost 500 million users worldwide, and it is still growing.[18] Will Twitter soon be an essential tool for medical practices?

More doctors are using Twitter to connect both with patients and other medical professionals. Some doctors simply do not have enough time to use Twitter. Furthermore, time spent with patients in the social media sphere is certainly not compensated by health insurance. But Twitter is an advantageous way to reach thousands of people at once. For busy doctors who often need to both inform patients and connect with other medical colleagues, that capability can be an invaluable.

Some hospitals have "live-tweeted" surgery to great fanfare, allowing the public a peek into the operating room and giving people an opportunity to ask the surgeons questions mid-procedure.

In early 2012, a hospital in Texas broadcasted an open heart surgery procedure live on Twitter, as shown in Figure 4.10. Before I go on, I'm not advocating that all doctors should be broadcasting their procedures live on the Web. This case involved a motivated hospital and surgeon, a relatively routine operation, and a patient who obviously agreed to have his surgery publicized.

Picture this scenario. Two physicians were in the operating room. The cardiothoracic surgeon who was using a headset video camera was able to take pictures and video of the operating field. Another doctor had a laptop, and was able to engage patients and answer questions on Twitter. Of course, the hospital was happy with the social media outcome, as the event generated more than 125 million impressions on Twitter and its affiliated platforms.

But the doctors involved were happy with the process and the results as well. When they were interviewed after the event, they explained how they were able to engage with millions of patients who were interested in open heart surgery by educating them, pulling the curtain back, and giving a peek into the operating room. Only a real-time platform like Twitter was able to offer that opportunity.

Data on current physician use of Twitter are scarce. A site called TwitterDoctors.net describes itself as "a directory of the most influential doctors on Twitter, updated hourly." This site lists nearly 1200 doctors, a very small number when you consider that

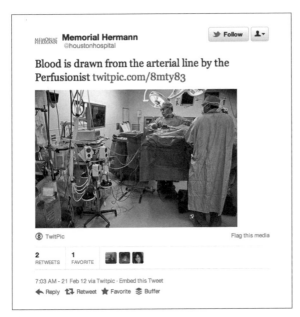

Memorial Hermann
@houstonhospital

Follow

Blood is drawn from the arterial line by the Perfusionist twitpic.com/8mty83

TwitPic   Flag this media

2   1
RETWEETS   FAVORITE

7:03 AM - 21 Feb 12 via Twitpic · Embed this Tweet
Reply Retweet Favorite Buffer

Figure 4.10

the total number of doctors in the United States alone is over 700,000.[19]

In 2011, Kathleen Chretien, MD, and colleagues from Washington, DC, published a study in the *Journal of the American Medical Association* describing the characteristics of physicians on Twitter and how they use it. Utilizing a rigorous process of excluding anyone with fewer than 500 followers and those who had not tweeted recently, the authors came up with 260 physicians they identified from public profile pages during the month of May 2010. The authors analyzed 5156 tweets by these physicians and found that 49% of the tweets were medical- and health related.[20] Given the number of tweets sent daily (more than 340 million in 2012), this finding indicates that physicians are definitely distributing a great deal of health information to the public.

The study found that 12% of the tweets were self-promotional. The authors also noted some unprofessional content and ethical violations such as profanity and patient privacy violations, but these occurrences were rare. Only 3% of all tweets were considered unprofessional. (The remainder were either personal communications or retweets.)[20] The goal, of course, is to have zero occurrences of unprofessional conduct. But there are no classes in medical school to teach students how to properly use social media. Few role models exist for young physicians today. The authors concluded that future education and guidelines may be needed to maximize the societal benefit of using Twitter. In the meantime, note the guidelines in the box Tips for Using Twitter Responsibly on page 86.

As medical student Michael Moore found out, the speed at which Twitter operates has an almost instant impact on a doctor's online reputation:

When it comes to online reputation, it is hard for me to think of an epiphany that really made me think of "managing" my online reputation.

If I had to point to just one "eureka" moment regarding the impact and importance of online reputation, it would have to be the beginning of my third year of medical school during the first week of my rotation. My role blogging for *The Lancet* had been publicized by the local medical community and the hospital that sponsored my university's students. As part of that publicity, my Twitter account was shared.

All of that was fine; my account is a great reflection of my personality (warts and all), and I am quite proud of the quality of my interaction there. However, an administrator came up to me and mentioned that an anonymous "physician" Twitter account that is quite caustic in its criticism of patients was publicly associated with me. He assumed that all physicians and medical students on Twitter would be critical of patients in that way.

I realized then that, in a way, for better or worse, we all share each other's reputation, a group identity, in the public eye.

Michael Moore
Medical Student
Yakima, Washington
www.thelancetstudent.com

Connect with Patients

Twitter offers a variety of ways for doctors to engage patients online. Ideally, the most useful tweets are those that provide commentary on medical news, to give it context and help patients understand what they are seeing and reading in the news media, or to keep them abreast of dynamically changing health situations.

During the H1N1 pandemic in the spring of 2009 for instance, people were panicked about the impact of the virus. My office was flooded with calls from worried patients.

TIPS FOR USING TWITTER RESPONSIBLY

1. Patient privacy must be maintained. Do not discuss specific cases or provide patient advice via Twitter.
2. Remember the "elevator test"—don't communicate anything over Twitter that you would not want overheard in a crowded hospital elevator.
3. Use Twitter to direct your patients to trustworthy online health information sources.
4. Remind patients using Twitter to be careful about who they follow. Make sure the person they are following is really a healthcare professional.
5. Use Twitter to promote your practice's brand. Patients are using Twitter and are likely to feel positive about their physicians using it as well.

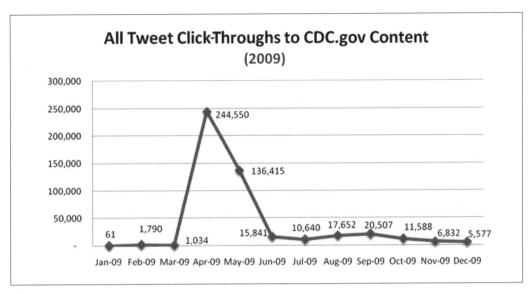

Figure 4.11

I directed some of them to the Twitter feed from the CDC, which provided up-to-the minute information on the status of the virus, as well as the vaccine.[21]

As you can see from Figure 4.11, during that time, that Twitter feed drove a significant amount of traffic to the CDC's website, where patients could read more detailed updates about the pandemic.

Otolaryngologist Bobby Ghaheri, MD, describes how Twitter better connects him with patients.

Twitter offers me a unique platform that I may use to connect with patients. I use it as a virtual office location. While making personal connections with potential patients sounds daunting, it is actually a very natural process. To many, the idea of seeing a new doctor is intimidating, especially in the context of seeing a surgical specialist.

Enter Twitter, where I maintain a constant presence. While I use it for my entertainment and personal connections with friends and family, I also use my Twitter account to serve as a dynamic resource for people in my city in addition to people around the world. I have many patients that I first met on Twitter, then later met in one of my terrestrial offices. The outcome: major surgeries for some (parotid, thyroid, and sinus) in addition to more routine cases (tonsillectomy, ear tubes, and scar revisions) for others. Office visits regarding management of seasonal allergies and hearing loss are also common.

People use Twitter to meet me and my personality (as I don't distinguish my actions on Twitter from my real-life persona). If they interact with me enough, they see who I am and what I'm about. This dramatically decreases the tension surrounding a potential office visit, which is most noticeable in the cosmetic arena. With frequent media focus surrounding negative outcomes from cosmetic procedures, patients can be quite hesitant to try an elective cosmetic procedure. With my online presence, that hesitancy decreases tremendously.

As an online office location, prospective patients can ask me questions (sometimes anonymously) at any time of the day. They get a personalized answer quickly and are grateful for the attention. I have found that the interactions on Twitter are more natural and personable than those on question-and-answer medical websites. I have personally chosen not to involve Facebook as I see that as a platform for my personal life. Where Twitter is concerned, however, the public nature allows me to connect with those who might never see me—across the city in addition to other states.

The majority of physicians still won't adopt a social media presence for quite some time. They worry about HIPAA (I'm careful not to discuss medical issues with existing patients) and litigation (I have a clearly defined social media policy). If doctors can get past those fears, the potential upside is tremendous. In this sense, doctors are really no different from any other professionals and should embrace the connections available to them.

Bobby Ghaheri, MD
Otolaryngologist
Portland, Oregon
http://wrinklewhisperer.squarespace.com
https://twitter.com/drghaheri

Connect with Other Healthcare Professionals

Twitter offers an invaluable opportunity for doctors to ask questions of other medical providers. Given the real-time nature of Twitter, opinions and answers to clinical issues can be obtained immediately. Healthcare professionals can also use it as a vehicle to break news ahead of the media, by tweeting important breakthroughs as they are announced at medical conferences.

As a busy primary care physician, I'm not able to attend as many conferences as I would like. And without live video or media coverage, there is no way for non-attendees to know what's happening during these conferences.

Increasingly, individuals are using their mobile devices or laptops to provide live Twitter updates of speakers as they are presenting. By following such a stream on Twitter, I am able to remotely "listen" to these speakers live. Of course, it doesn't replace actually being there, but without Twitter, I would have missed many key presentations over the years.

Christian Sinclair, MD, a palliative care physician, explains how Twitter can be used at medical conferences[22]:

The growing field of palliative medicine has a strong social media presence, and the addition of more people into our online network helps get important information to people far beyond the patients and families we see each day in our work.

Twitter can be a great way to capture the small nuggets of information you glean while at a conference. Don't worry about trying to post everything from a single slide, but try to find the fact or theme that resonates with you. Hopefully your speaker actually included the slides for you to reference later or, even better, posted them online via Slideshare or Scribd so you can access them anytime. After the conference, you can look back through your stream of posts and see a record of what you found inspiring. And as a bonus, you can see what other people retweeted, which may further reinforce what is really important. Also, if you are planning on posting copiously from a lecture, make sure to include the last name of the speaker on each post so that he or she is correctly cited.

Twitter as Conversation Starter

While you are posting about an interesting point, people at the conference and those not at the conference may find that point interesting and may ask you a question and engage you in further discussion. I have had situations where people (not at the conference) asked me questions that I later asked the speaker. Many times the people I am posting with during a conference are people that I want to seek out and talk to in person, a good example of online engagement becoming offline action.

Twitter as Feedback Monitor

Are you a speaker at a conference with a good social media presence? You might want to check the feed for your name and presentation. I recall one presentation where everyone online started reporting an inability to read any of the slides. Some people then posted the slides online for all to see.

For a speaker, this is not good presenting. And Twitter may help you avoid a problem in the future.

Twitter as Influence Generator

If you are a power user of Twitter, you may be able to create expanding waves of influence through original posts and selective retweeting at a medical conference. This can also work if you are not at the conference but the topic resonates with you. One interesting paradox with Twitter is the more you post, the more people will follow you. A few people will drop off, but if you post a few warnings that this is an intense period of tweeting on a focused subject, many more will stick around. Being influential is also very possible if you are already influential offline. Just being on Twitter and posting four to five tweets per day as an important offline persona can be a great addition to a conference.

Twitter as Event Planner

If you start tweeting at a conference, chances are you are going to find other like-minded people that you may decide to meet in person. Congratulations, you will have participated in a "tweetup"! Twitter can also be a quick way to find out what is going on at a medical conference that you may be interested in since the organization and exhibitors may be posting events.

Twitter as Goodwill Creator

Maybe you don't want to be burdened with writing original posts, but you can still be part of the wave of influence by retweeting other people's great posts. In sharing other people's posts, you are basically complimenting the other person, which makes the original poster happy, and other people will not think you are a selfish egoist who cares only about your own thoughts. Besides, social media is essentially about sharing, right?

Twitter as Impact Maker

Have 10,000 followers on Twitter? One or two posts from a medical conference may point hundreds of people to information they never would have sought on their own. For what was only a few seconds of your time, you will have helped grow a community and connected people with similar interests. Personally I would be happy to post about any medical conference to my network, just ask.

Christian T. Sinclair, MD, FAAHPM

Palliative Care Physician
Overland Park, Kansas
www.pallimed.org

Essentials

If you have never used Twitter before and terms like "tweet" and "hashtag" sound foreign to you, you should spend some time exploring the site. Twitter is a real-time information network, and if you carefully choose people to follow, you'll have access to the latest news, opinions, and thoughts on any topic you find interesting.

Step 1. Search without signing up. If you are completely unfamiliar with Twitter and are reluctant to set up an account just yet, you can explore the site first, without creating an account. To do so, go to http://search.twitter.com and enter a few keywords to see relevant recent tweets. You can search a medical specialty, an organization or person's name, or any keyword of a topic that interests you. Nearly all medical societies, as well as most medical journals, have Twitter accounts. The homepage of the society or journal is likely to have a Twitter icon you can simply click to "follow" it. You can also see who *it* follows and will probably find other organizations or people with common interests. You can also just see what kinds of conversations are happening right now. If you want to monitor for updates on Twitter, you can set up a Google Alert. For example, you could decide to be e-mailed by Google Alerts every time it indexes a tweet mentioning skin cancer, using this search: "site:twitter.com skin cancer."

Step 2. Make an account. Go to https://twitter.com/signup and enter your desired username and password and your e-mail address. Your username should be your real name. Remember, you are doing this to further your online reputation and have your name appear higher in search results, so it is important to remain consistent in social media by using the same name on all of your sites. If your chosen username is already taken, the site will give you other options (such as numbers added after your name) or you can append some other relevant descriptor, such as your specialty. Example: Susan_SmithPeds.

Step 3. Find people to follow. After signing up, Twitter will take you through a series of actions to select people to follow and start building your network. You can find people through keyword searches or the site will suggest potential related connections. Select well-known physicians or other leaders you admire, then colleagues you know and respect. The site will ask to check your e-mail to find connections already on Twitter. (Twitter clearly states that it does not use or share this information; it's just a shortcut to help you identify people you might like to follow.) By following people, you'll be able to see what they think is important and find links to interesting articles. If you choose people to follow wisely, you may find that Twitter gives you a great deal of valuable, real-time information you would not get elsewhere. You can then choose to comment on a noteworthy tweet or perhaps retweet it with your followers.

Step 4. Add to your profile. Once you've selected some people to follow, you are directed to the Profile page. You can skip directly to this page if you prefer and set up your profile first. Here you are given an opportunity to brand yourself and your practice on Twitter. You can add a profile picture, your name, location, website, and a short bio (160 characters or less). The bio can be similar to your Facebook or LinkedIn bio. In fact, some experts recommend that you use some of the same wording—even cut and paste—from bios elsewhere so that your branding is consistent across various social media sites. There is also Facebook integration; with this feature, you can have tweets you send on Twitter posted on your Facebook page at the same time.

Step 5. Tweet! If you decide that you want your voice heard in the Twitterverse, you can also do this in an incremental fashion. You can "try out" using Twitter before deciding to become an active participant by making your account private. Go to the Account page, and under "Tweet Privacy" check the box next to "Protect my Tweets." Any tweets you create will be sent only to people you have specifically authorized. Tweets appear in reverse chronological order, with the most recent being on top of the list in your Twitter feed.

While the maximum length of a tweet is 140 characters, experts advise that you try to limit your tweets to about 120 characters, including spaces, punctuation, and URLs. This will make it easier for your followers to retweet a message you post without having to shorten it.

It might take some time to master the art of tweeting, to make the most out of that character limit. Abbreviations are commonly used to keep character counts down. For example, "pls" for "please" and "msg" for "message" are two such abbreviations. Other techniques for saving characters include: dropping vowels ("jrnl" for "journal"); using numerals ("3" not "three"); and omitting unnecessary words ("+" instead of "and"). Forget everything you learned about formal writing. The goal is to communicate effectively in as few words as possible.

Maximizing Twitter

Get people to follow you. The best way to maximize your presence on Twitter is to get followers. Just following other people will not boost your reputation on Twitter. You need to give others a reason to follow *you.* You can build a following simply by tweeting and retweeting interesting news updates. Contribute to the conversation by talking about issues that are really important to your audience, and watch the number of your followers grow!

You can also invite followers from your practice by putting a notice in your office and on your website promoting your presence on Twitter. The more people who follow you, the more other people will want to follow you because you will be considered an influential voice in the field.

Listen and learn. Twitter is a tremendous way to filter the vast amounts of information on the Web. Once you have found several people with common interests to follow on Twitter, you can add them to a list, and simply listen to what they have to say and read the articles that they share. It's like having a personal concierge picking the best articles on the Web for you to read.

Promote yourself. You can also promote your presence on Twitter by linking it to your LinkedIn profile and/or your Facebook page. You should also add a Twitter icon like 🐦 or 🄱 to your website and include a link to your Twitter page so that patients and others who visit your site can go directly to your Twitter site as well.

If you're not yet convinced of the powerful role that Twitter can play in healthcare, consider the following story from Edmond Kwok, MD, a Canadian emergency physician:

> It was my first ER shift in charge of the resuscitation area. Needless to say, my adrenaline and nerves were firing like crazy; being responsible for the sickest of the sick that roll through our doors is a daunting task, especially since we were the local trauma center. The shift was going relatively well; and with only a few hours left, I was beginning to breathe a sigh of relief.
>
> *BEEP!*
>
> There is no mistaking that obnoxiously loud paramedic patch phone ring, even from the other end of the department. I turned and saw the charge nurse pick up the call. The knot in my stomach quickly tightened as I watched the color literally drain from her face, before she asked over the phone, "I'm sorry, *what?*"
>
> Oh, I had forgotten to mention, it was a July evening with the biggest annual outdoor music festival being hosted in our city. Apparently, a freak thunderstorm decided to pound its way through the city, and the main stage of the final act collapsed mid-act. The only information that was conveyed over the patch call before the paramedics rushed into the chaotic scene was this: "The main stage at Bluesfest collapsed on the crowd! Likely people

trapped under with penetrating wounds! No idea how many—expect the worst!"

One of the most important decisions for a receiving mass casualty facility to make in such a scenario is how to prepare adequately for the potentially overwhelming influx of critically ill patients. In Canada, most hospitals have structured contingency plans for this, commonly known as a Code Orange. It usually involves a rapid call-out to off-duty staff to come in, mobilization of patients out of the ER and into the hospital hallways, and canceling all elective surgeries and procedures.

Code Orange is a *very* expensive protocol and can negatively affect patients who are already in the hospital as we try to create surge capacity for mass casualty events. You might even remember stories of Code Orange being called for severe ER overcrowding. And the decision to trigger a Code Orange for the stage collapse? All mine.

The problem was, I felt like there just wasn't enough information to make that decision. Were we expecting 2 or 200 patients? Did they have serious wounds or minor scratches? How quickly would they be coming through our doors—all at once by ambulance, or slowly as they made their own way to the ER?

We tried calling the paramedics back, but no luck. They, of course, were busy at the scene. Then I heard a resident beside me wonder out loud as she pulled out her iPhone, "Hmm, I wonder what people there are tweeting."

I paused. Tweeting? Isn't that some weird online blogging thing?

We quickly logged onto Twitter, and found a steady stream of live updates from spectators at the scene.

Wow, main stage collapsed, while the band was still on!

Giant storm hits Bluesfest! Stage down! Everyone running—but no one hurt?

Paramedics searching . . . no one seems hurt!

I was getting much more accurate up-to-the-second information on what was going on through the many eyes of the Twitter users than I was getting from official paramedic and police channels. It was the first time I caught a glimpse of what a powerful tool social media could potentially be in healthcare, despite all the press on the concerns regarding confidentiality, reliability of medical information, and lack of regulation.

How do you see the evolution of social media in your healthcare?

Edmund Kwok, MD
Emergency Medicine Physician
Ottawa, Ontario, Canada
http://frontdoor2healthcare.wordpress.com

TWITTER LINGO

There are some symbols and naming conventions used in Twitter that you will need to know to effectively use the site. Below are explanations and examples of the major ones.

@ (example: @kevinmd): This is your username. It appears when you are referring directly to or about a user. So, for example, when you reply to a specific user by clicking the Reply button under his or her tweet, that user's @name will automatically appear at the beginning of your tweet. If you are not replying but want to mention a specific user, you would first put the symbol @, then the person's username. (See Figure 4.12.)

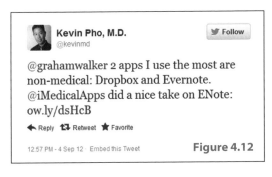

Figure 4.12

 # (Hashtag): The # symbol is not called the pound sign but rather a hashtag. It is used to mark keywords or topics in a tweet. You should use the hashtag symbol # before a relevant keyword or phrase (no spaces) in a tweet to categorize those tweets and help them show more easily in a Twitter search. If you click on a word with a hashtag in any message, you can see all other tweets marked with that keyword. Hashtags can be placed anywhere in the tweet—at the beginning, middle, or end. (See Figure 4.13.)

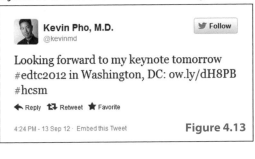

Figure 4.13

(RT) (Retweet): A retweet is a reposting of someone else's tweet. This feature helps you and others quickly share that tweet with all of your followers. Retweets look like normal tweets with the author's name and username next to it, but are **distinguished by the retweet icon** and the name of the user who retweeted the tweet. If you see a message from a stranger in your timeline, it was probably retweeted by someone you follow. (See Figure 4.14.)

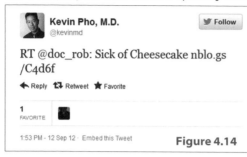

Figure 4.14

(MT) (Modified tweet): This abbreviation is often used when someone retweets a post but needs to edit or modify it in some way to fit his or her own comment and the original tweet into the maximum allowance of 140 characters. (See Figure 4.15.)

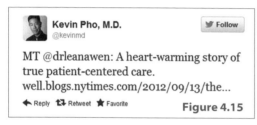

Figure 4.15

(DM) (Direct message): If you want to send a private message to one of your followers, use this feature. You can send a direct message only to someone who is following you, and you can receive direct messages only from people you follow.

Unfamiliar links in a tweet: Have you ever noticed an odd-looking link in a tweet? Here's an example from a recent American Academy of Pediatrics tweet:

> Today in Pediatrics: Infants born at 37 or 38 weeks have lower test scores in 3rd grade http://ow.ly/bXDDS

This tweet includes a shortened link. Clicking on it will take you to a Web page whose link has specifically been shortened to fit into a tweet. The original article link looked like this:

> www.aap.org/en-us/about-the-aap/aap-press-room/pages/Infants-Born-at-37-or-38-weeks-have-Increased-Risk-of-Lower-Test-Scores-in-Third-Grade.aspx.

This link exceeds the maximum character allowance for a tweet and, of course, would not allow room for comment even if were a few words shorter. There are external sites that will make these conversions for you, and when you include links in you tweets, Twitter will shorten them for you.

Follow: Clicking the Follow button on the Twitter page of a person or an organization allows you to subscribe to the updates of that person or group. The total number of people you follow will appear under "Following" in your Twitter profile.

Follower: The people who have signed up to follow you on Twitter.

BLOGS: YOUR SOCIAL MEDIA HUB

Blogs are short for "web logs," defined by Wikipedia as "a website where entries are written in chronological order and commonly displayed in reverse chronological order."[23]

In its simplest form, a blog is an online diary (see Figure 4.16). Blogs are highly personal in nature and design. All of the blogs together with the links connecting them are referred to as the "blogosphere." Like fingerprints and snowflakes, no two blogs are exactly alike. Creating a blog gives you a chance to build something that is a unique reflection of you.

Originally used by computer professionals, the popularity of blogs has grown widely over the past decade. By the end of 2011, there had been an explosive growth in the number of blogs. NM Incite, a Nielson/McKinsey company, tracked 181 million blogs,

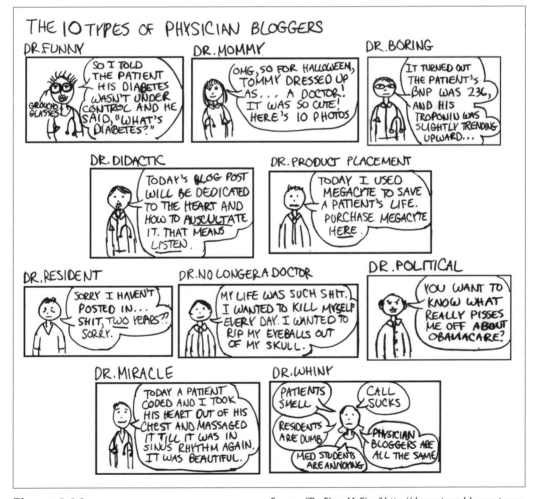

Figure 4.16   Source: "Dr. Fizzy McFizz," http://doccartoon.blogspot.com.

up from *just* 36 million in 2006.[24] The WordPress.com platform alone accounts for more than 57 million blogs.[25]

There have been few scientific studies or journal reports about medical and healthcare blogs. In 2008, two Canadian authors addressed this topic and implored physicians "Don't Do It."[26] That same year, authors from Croatia reported results of a survey of medical bloggers. Responses from 80 English-language medical bloggers showed them to be highly educated and devoted blog writers who were motivated to share practical knowledge, influence the way people think, and express themselves creatively.[27]

Medical and healthcare blogs are quite diverse. Organizations and commercial companies often have a blog associated with their website to highlight new products or services, while individuals tell stories and offer opinions. You may be wondering what new information could possibly be added to the blogosphere.

All of the stories featured in this book come from people—both physicians and patients—who actively blog. Their reasons for doing so are as diverse as the fields they represent or the conditions they have, but they do have some common characteristics.

Physicians blog because they want to share important and evidence-based healthcare information with patients and the community. They have knowledge and expertise and want to be an authoritative voice in the blogosphere. They want to guide their patients to other quality sources of health information. Some want patients to know more about the healthcare system and changes in health policy. In other words, they want to educate and engage patients. They want to make a difference in patients' lives.

Patients, on the other hand, blog to share their stories and write about their experiences. Physicians can learn a tremendous amount from reading patients' viewpoints, as most don't know what it's like to be a patient today in our healthcare system.

Blogs offer two key advantages over some other types of social media. First, they rank high in search engine result pages. Recently, Google made changes to its search algorithms that have an even more positive effect on blogs. Google's Panda update looks at the quality of the content and penalizes the exploitation of keywords. So if a marketing consultant has encouraged you to put a large number of keywords on your website without real content to back them up, you may find your site drops in search engine rankings. Google's Penguin update looks for unnatural links. But if you link to other credible sources, you'll come out ahead. Now more than ever, a blog allows you to post updated content that appeals to the search engines.

Second, you have more control over your content. On Twitter and Facebook, your content is subject to the whims of their constantly changing terms and conditions. If Facebook wants to inject more advertisements into your wall, for instance, there's little you can do about it. On a blog, however, how you shape your content is entirely up to you.

It makes sense to have a blog be your social media hub, as I do with KevinMD.com. Complementary platforms like Twitter, LinkedIn, Facebook, and Google+ can then be your social media spokes, where you can attract patients who consume information and engage on different social media sites.

Internal medicine physician John Schumann, MD, reflects on how his blog gives him a platform to share his thoughts and increases his influence through attention from mainstream media:

> For years, Internet-savvy friends encouraged me to start a blog as a way of communicating medical topics to non-medical readers.
>
> "What interesting or novel things do I have to say?," I always countered. "Who would read such a blog?" I pronounced the word "blog" with a nasal inflection, showing my distaste for the trendy new Internet-influenced word.
>
> I only wish I'd listened sooner.
>
> After practicing medicine for more than a decade, I've stored up a lot of things that I want to say about how medicine *is* practiced and how it *should be* practiced. Sometimes, my opinions ruffle feathers, though I never aim to do that. I'm aiming for the sweet spot between educating and entertaining readers. The insatiable appetite for medical news and information has made it all the more imperative to have thoughtful, responsible voices in the blogosphere (a term I now embrace) and writing for mainstream publications (which I've now had the opportunity to do).
>
> Within eight months of starting a regular weekly medical blog, Glass Hospital.com, I was published in a national magazine, written about in a major newspaper for crowdsourcing a diagnosis, and invited to contribute advice to an Internet startup looking for best practices in electronic doctor-patient communication.
>
> All because I was willing to put my ideas out into cyberspace.
>
> My online reputation is very important to me. As an academic physician without a traditional research portfolio to fall back on, social media has become a distinct tool for peer-to-peer networking and even academic promotion. My "authority" as a medical pundit stems from the serious

topics that I tackle (suffering, death, health policy, and patient experiences) on my blog, and now via Facebook and Twitter.

I was slow to adopt social networking sites to communicate medical topics, just like I was with starting a blog. It's a crowded space that seems to become more so all the time—thus there's no time like right now to start "hanging your shingle" out there in cyberspace.

My online activities have brought me "traditional" medical business, though that's not a goal of my writing. Nevertheless, I always feel good when someone seeks me out because of something that I've written.

John Schumann, MD
Internal Medicine Physician
Associate Director, Internal Medicine Residency Program
University of Oklahoma School of Community Medicine
Tulsa, Oklahoma
http://glasshospital.com

Essentials

The mechanics of creating a blog are quite easy. Blog-hosting sites today have created tools so that anyone with basic computer skills can start a blog in minutes. The hard work comes in setting goals and writing the content.

Step 1. Do your due diligence. If you don't currently follow any blogs in your field, search for blogs on topics that interest you or are relevant to your practice and your field. Chances are you will find hundreds or millions of blogs and blog posts in your initial search. For example, a search for "sports medicine" turned up over 22 million blog results on Google. You can refine your search, depending on the search engine you use.

Step 2. Determine the goals and scope for your blog. Think about the kinds of information you talk or write about on a regular basis. Your blog could either be focused on a theme or it could be a blog that provides links and commentary to interesting new sites, or a mixture of the two. Be careful to identify your goals, and then stick to them.

If your blog is intended for patients, make sure you write about the topics they are interested in. Start by asking patients what kind of information they would find most helpful, then use their responses to develop your topic list. Once your blog is published and active, you can start directing patients there as an educational service.

Step 3. Choose a name. The name of your blog is a key to its visibility in search engine results because they will pick up the title as keywords. You might want to include your practice name or geographic location (for example, Seattle Mama Doc, or KC Kids Doc). The title of your blog doesn't have to be the username you created for the account, but can be a descriptive or catchy name.

Whatever blog name you choose, best practices suggest that you should post under your own name. You can only be truly authoritative if you publish in your own name, and there is no way to build your online reputation unless you do.

Step 4. Choose a platform. There are several free platforms available for building your blog. I recommend Blogger, WordPress, or Tumblr. Blogger, formerly known as Blogspot, is now owned by Google. With your Google account, you can create as many blogs as you like on Blogger.

Blogger, WordPress, and Tumblr have similar steps to follow in creating your blog. They are intuitive and will help you create a blog in as little as five minutes. Each is hosted on its own server.

Your new blog will be given a custom link. Since there are already a large number of blogs in existence, you may have to try a few different names before you find one that is available.

The format for your link on Blogger will be [yoursite].blogspot.com. For WordPress, the link will be [yoursite].wordpress.com. And for Tumblr, the link will be [yoursite].tumblr.com.

Each platform gives you the option of mapping your given domain to a custom one (for example, [yoursite].wordpress.com to www.[yoursite].com). Although not essential, I recommend taking this additional step. Doing so clarifies your online brand.

For advanced bloggers, WordPress can be hosted on the blogger's own server for greater control and flexibility. The advantage is that the blogger totally owns his or her content, meaning the information is stored on servers the blogger controls, rather than those owned by a third party. That's also a disadvantage, since administering a server requires time, money, and effort, which many providers don't have. So for the sake of this chapter, which focuses on fast, free ways to build a digital footprint, I'm not going to provide more detail about this path.

Which platform should you choose? If you regularly write longer posts, say over 500 words, WordPress and Blogger are better suited to long-form blogs. If your posts are short and pithy, you link to a lot of interesting sites, or simply post pictures and video without much accompanying text, Tumblr is a better fit. In fact, some consider Tumblr a "tweener" platform: in between Twitter and blogs.

After signing up to your platform of choice, you will be taken to a dashboard, or control center, for your blog. Here you can control many aspects of your blog's function, design, and appearance. Follow the instructions, and customize your blog by looking at different templates, themes, and designs. For example, you could link to other relevant sites to provide more information on the topic you are posting about or add information from your practice, like a registration form or an appointment scheduler.

Step 5. Start writing. I started KevinMD.com in 2004, when blogging was in its infancy. Since then, a continual complaint I've heard from many healthcare providers is that writing regularly can be a challenge. Here are some tips that I'd like to share, both from myself and other blog experts:

Imagine that you're talking to a friend. I find the best blogs tend to be informal and approachable. The best way to accomplish such a tone is to be conversational. Marc Ambinder, contributing editor at *The Atlantic*, shares this blogging pearl: "I've found that I tend to write the way I speak. Short, staccato sentences, lots of parentheticals. That annoys purists, but it's uniquely my own voice, and I think it helps to build a connection with the reader."[28]

Think about your audience. Are you talking to patients? Then be sure to write in a casual manner, and explain medical jargon, or avoid it altogether. Is your audience primarily doctors? Then you can include more arcane terms or lingo that only medical professionals may know, or tackle physician-specific topics.

Focus on the theme of your blog. As you develop your blog further by posting regular articles, you will need to organize your posts by genre and category to reflect the keywords in your articles and make it easier for people to find your posts. On KevinMD. com, I categorize posts by topic: physician opinion, patient specific, social media tutorials, medical technology, health news, medical education, and healthcare policy.

Posts should be at least 300 words. Search engines place less weight on articles shorter than that. Of course, blogs can be as long as you want, but keep in mind the attention span of a typical Internet user, who may not have time to sit in front of a computer and read feature-length essays. Editors at the Huffington Post recommend that posts be no longer than 800 words.[29] I aim for between 500 and 1000 words on my posts.

Don't worry if your posts aren't perfect. Aiming for every post to be a literary masterpiece simply isn't sustainable for most blogs. Make sure the spelling and grammar are correct, but don't worry if the final product won't win a Pulitzer. Felix Salmon, who writes *Portfolio*'s finance blog Market Movers, says to blogging beginners, "Don't be scared of being wrong, or inelegant; you have much less of an idea what your readers are going to like than you possibly imagine. So jump right in, put yourself out there."[28]

Post according to a schedule. It could range from several times a week to every day. The Huffington Post editors say, "If you're serious about blogging, commit to posting at least two to three times a week for thirty days."[29] That may seem daunting to the typical healthcare professional, but a blog is only as good as the time spent on it. The more regularly you write, the more readers will come back knowing there will be more.

Pay attention to the title. This is arguably the most important part of your posts. Darren Rowse, who founded the popular how-to blogging site ProBlogger, proclaims that, "Titles change the destiny of your posts."[30] He's absolutely right. People often decide whether or not to read your article based solely on its title.

Furthermore, those blog titles will appear throughout the Web on RSS feeds, other social media sites, links from other bloggers, and most importantly, on search engines. When your blog is indexed on Google, it's the title that most people read (see Figure 4.17).

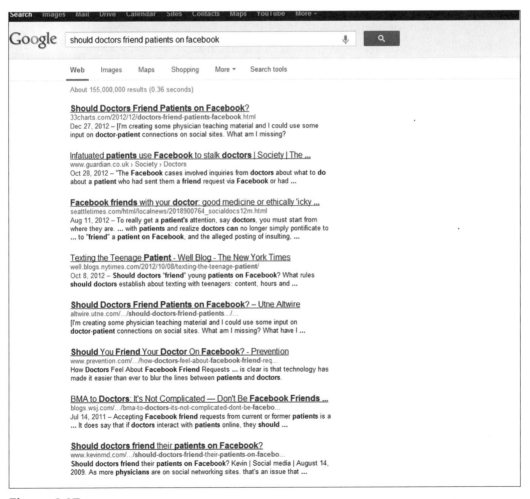

Figure 4.17

There are many approaches to crafting a blog title, which can by themselves be a chapter of a book. Keep titles shorter than 70 characters (because that's about the maximum length Google shows on its result pages), and mix in different title styles. Here are some titles that resonate, with examples of actual ones that I've used in my own blog:

- **Show a benefit**
  - Three unexpected ways to help you lose weight
  - Why going to a board-certified plastic surgeon is important
  - Ten tips for new college students with chronic disease
- **Ask a question**
  - Are Medicare vouchers a good idea for patients and their physicians?
  - Can the airline industry teach customer service lessons to medicine?
  - Why do patients often deviate from their advance directives?
- **Be provocative**
  - Why I want to ration your health care
  - Why one-third of hospitals will close by 2020
  - Granting rights to a fetus at the cost of the mother
- **Make it personal**
  - I learn from patients who share their stories on Twitter
  - I have seen the tragedy of prescription drug abuse
  - As I reach the end of my career, I empathize more with my patients

Maximizing Blogs

Find the time to blog. While writing regular blog posts takes discipline, it doesn't have to be burdensome. Howard Luks, MD, orthopedist and social media consultant, shares how he maintains his blog while also regularly seeing patients:

> **Think of blogging as your 21st, or 41st, or 51st patient.**
>
> **Our workflow is simple. We dictate. We dictate every single note about every single patient at the end of each and every visit. We say a lot of the same things each and every day. That is content. That is important, meaningful content that patients will find useful.**
>
> **Let your patients drive your content management strategy. Patients are the ones who are suffering—that bring up questions and searches. Patients are the ones who are searching online—yet still have questions. Those patients are asking you the same questions every day.**
>
> **Write them down!**

Let's say your day is done and you are sitting in your back office. Take out the list of questions, and go through the following steps:

- What are the most common questions that were asked? Those are the titles of your blog post.
- Pick up your Dictaphone, and dictate a few paragraphs to address the question.
- Transcribe the dictation by sending it to someone (or do the work yourself), and publish it on your blog.

Those five minutes of effort will pay off for years to come. When you have mastered this and it becomes an efficient, smooth part of your workflow, you will find that your presence will be most visible online.

Eventually, the Google rank of these blog posts will rise and further boost your online presence.

Howard Luks, MD
Orthopedic Surgeon
Associate Professor of Orthopedic Surgery
New York Medical College
Hawthorne, New York
www.howardluksmd.com

Measure blog statistics. Want to know who's been reading your blog? Blogger and Tumblr allow you to install Google Analytics, a free tool that provides a detailed analysis of your audience, including the number of visitors, hits, and page views for your blog. WordPress has analytics built in.

You can find out which sites, blogs, or social media platforms are sending people your way. If you get a surge of traffic from a specific source, be sure to thank that source via an e-mail, through your blog, or on Twitter or Facebook.

By reviewing the list of keywords and keyword phrases in the statistics, you can learn what keywords people used in their searches that led them to you. You can even see how much of your audience is accessing your blog through mobile devices or a desktop computer.

Using analytics can also fine-tune your topics. For instance, if a post is particularly popular, be sure to keep it updated to ensure people continue to read the latest information. Or if readers are finding your site using specific keywords, write more posts related to those topics.

Be patient. This is perhaps the most critical point. It takes time to build a following, especially with the millions of voices already on the blogosphere today. Wait a year, at least. Slowly, people will start to pay attention. Tens of readers will turn into hundreds, and those hundreds into thousands.

And remember, there are reasons for blogging other than gaining readership. For me, blogging has sharpened my writing and helped me to clarify my thoughts on a particular subject. I've also put my personal stamp on the Web, and who knows which patient I've reached through a blog post that he or she found via Google.

GOOGLE: MAPPING THE FUTURE

Google's offerings in social media are quickly changing, and doctors cannot afford to ignore them. A major reason for its importance is because, well, it's Google—so you can expect any social media tools it creates to figure prominently in searches. In the past few years, Google has added features that you can use to create a visible online profile, enhance your online business listing, and share information with others. It's not just a search engine any more.

Google had made previous forays into the social media space, but it has been most successful with Google+ (pronounced and sometimes written as "Google-Plus"), which was introduced in 2011. It's also seen sometimes just a "g+" or "G+." A social networking and identity service, Google+ has 400 million registered users as of September 2012, 100 million of whom are active every month.[31] Google+ incorporates profiles and also includes services called Circles and Hangouts, all built to facilitate users' ability to organize their contacts into groups for communicating and sharing updates, news stories, and other information of mutual interest. Google Places pages were created for businesses, a concept similar to Facebook pages. Significant changes were made in the summer of 2012 when Google Places was replaced with Google+ Local.

Given Google's increasing prominence in social media, you may wonder why we have chosen to discuss it last in the chapter on defining your online identity. The answer lies in the hybrid nature of the site. You can create a profile on Google+. That profile will be displayed in Google results when people search for your name. Thus, it's a key component of the online identity you create for yourself.

In addition to the personal profile, you can create a dynamic Google+ Local page with pertinent details (to which Google will add a map) to help patients find you. You can also correct any errors in the listing Google has for your practice.

Beyond those basic building blocks, the most recent changes have profound implications for medical practices. Google is actively integrating Google+ Local across its other properties. One key part of the plan involves adding a review component to *every* Google+ Local listing. Many Google+ Local listings already contain links to reviews on major rating sites, such as Vitals.

In fact, it is this hybrid nature of Google+ Local that makes it difficult to place in this book. As it builds its own rating system, Google+ Local may be more akin to the rating sites in the future. Yet it's a fundamental strategic site where you want to take control of how your name and practice appear, and it is integral to other tools you may be using such as Blogger and YouTube. Thus, addressing Google here allows us to concentrate on guidelines for creating a good profile that will enhance your digital footprint; and, in the next chapter, your Google+ Local page and the associated rating system will be further explored.

Essentials

Step 1. Create an account. To get started with all things Google, you must first create an account. On the Google homepage, www.google.com, you select "Sign In," or if you do not yet have an account, the upper right corner of the page includes a red box for "Sign Up." You already have an account if you use YouTube or Google docs, or if you have a Gmail account. If you don't, it's a straightforward process. When you select "Sign Up," you are taken to the main Google account page. Simply supply the requested information, including a username and password, and you will soon have your account.

Step 2. Create a profile. When you sign into your account, you will be taken to the Google+ page, as shown in Figure 4.18. You'll have the option to learn more about Google+ by watching a video or you can begin creating your profile. To do so now or any time you come back to your page, simply click on your username at the top of your Google+ page after you sign in, and select "View Profile."

Click on the "About" tab, then "Edit profile," and a template will appear. You will be prompted to provide information on your education, employment, places you've lived, and other personal details. You're given the opportunity to come up with a unique tagline for yourself. Here are some examples:

- Howard Luks, MD: Orthopedic Surgeon, Digital Thinker, Adviser, Consultant;
- Natasha Burgert, MD: Wife, Mom, Pediatrician, Blogger;
- Bryan Vartabedian, MD: Freerange physician; and
- Nick Genes, MD: NYC emergency medicine doctor with an interest in informatics.

Other tabs are for posting updates, uploading photos or videos, or adding "+1's" (Google's equivalent of a Like button).

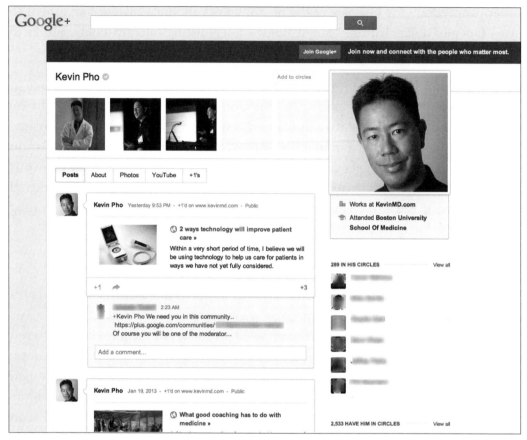

Figure 4.18

You can also choose to leave any of those fields blank. You can select who may see certain information about you. You can go to your dashboard at https://www.google.com/dashboard to manage personal data collected by Google across all of its sites. For maximum visibility in search results, your profile should be public; you will also want to link your website to it. Keep in mind that any public comments or posts on your Google+ page are indexed by search engines even if you have selected privacy settings for your personal information.

Maximizing Google+

Update and share. Even though the profile you created on Google+ is unique, the information was created using a template supplied by Google, which other people will use as well. To further customize your listing, post periodic updates. Share links to valuable information or articles that you come across. By creating fresh content on a regular basis, you can make your listing stand out from those of other practitioners in your area.

Link to your blog posts on Google+. This has three substantial benefits:

- Google has limited access to the data in Facebook and Twitter, meaning that those platforms have limited search engine optimization impact. Not so with Google+, where all of its data are available to Google. Google+ posts tend to rank higher when compared with competing posts from Twitter, Facebook, and LinkedIn.
- Google rapidly indexes content shared on Google+.
- As more people share the post, the value of the link increases, causing the blog post to rise in Google search results.

Link throughout your profile. Add links to your website and other social media profiles in the About page of your Google+ profile, specifically in the Introduction, Other profiles, and Links sections. Google+ will pass authority to those links, helping your other online presences rank higher in Google.

Organize your contacts. Circles are a key feature of Google+. According to Google, Circles allow you to "give and get updates from just the right people." What does this mean? When you add contacts on Google+, you have the opportunity place them in a "circle," or list. Sample circles can be "friends," "family," "acquaintances," or even "patients." You have the option to create customized circles (see Figure 4.19).

The ability to organize contacts is powerful. Healthcare providers need to be vigilant in using that feature.

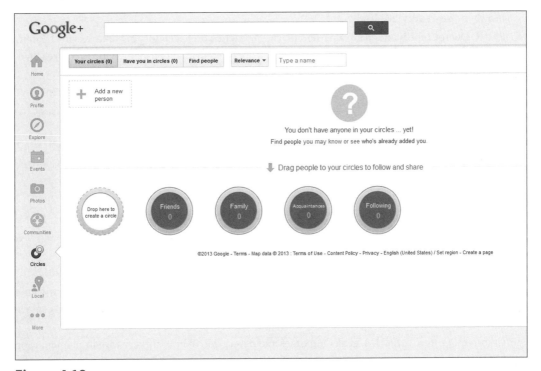

Figure 4.19

Most importantly, circles can have different news streams, meaning you can share information with selected groups of people. For instance, share physician-specific information with a colleagues circle and patient education material with a patients circle. This makes it easy to separate personal and professional content.

If Google+ ever reaches critical mass, it has potential to be *the* social network of choice for physicians. And circles will be the main reason why. ⁘

REFERENCES

1. Godin S. define: Brand. Seth Godin's Blog. http://sethgodin.typepad.com/seths_blog/2009/12/define-brand.html. Accessed November 12, 2012.

2. One Billion People on Facebook. Facebook Newsroom. http://newsroom.fb.com/News/One-Billion-People-on-Facebook-1c9.aspx. Accessed November 4, 2012.

3. 1 in 5 Americans Use Social Media for Health Care Information. Ticker. National Research Corporation. http://hcmg.nationalresearch.com/public/News.aspx?ID=9. Accessed November 5, 2012.

4. Fox S, Jones S. Social Life of Health Information. Pew Internet & American Life Project. 2009; www.pewinternet.org/Reports/2009/8-The-Social-Life-of-Health-Information/04-The-Social-Life-of-Health-Information/2-Social-networking-sites-are-used-only-sparingly-for-health-queries.aspx. Accessed November 7, 2012.

5. Greene JA, Choudhry NK, Kilabuk E, Shrank WH. Online social networking by patients with diabetes: a qualitative evaluation of communication with Facebook. *Journal Gen Intern Med*. 2011;26:287-292.

6. BUPA. Global Trends, Attitudes and Influences. 2011; www.bupa.com/media/288798/bupa_health_pulse_report_2011.pdf.

7. Pho K. Doctor reprimanded after patient privacy breached on Facebook, my take. KevinMD.com. April 20, 2011; www.kevinmd.com/blog/2011/04/doctor-reprimanded-patient-privacy-breached-facebook.html. Accessed November 7, 2012.

8. Mostaghimi A, Crotty BH. Professionalism in the digital age. *Ann Intern Med*. 2011;154:560-562.

9. Pediatric Associates Kansas City. Facebook. www.facebook.com/Pediatric.Associates.Kansas.City. Accessed November 7, 2012.

10. Baum N. How Often Do You Need to See Me? Dr. Neil Baum's Urology Blog. September 1, 2012; http://neilbaum.wordpress.com/2012/09/01/how-often-do-you-need-to-see-me. Accessed November 7, 2012.

11. Macarthur OB/GYN. Facebook. www.facebook.com/macobgyn. Accessed November 7, 2012.

12. Gordon D. YouTube: The Monster Search Engine You Can't Ignore. Search Insider blog, Media Post Publications. December 5, 2011; www.mediapost.com/publications/article/163492/youtube-the-monster-search-engine-you-cant-ignor.html. Accessed November 7, 2012.

13. YouTube. Press statistics. www.youtube.com/t/press_statistics. Accessed November 7, 2012.

14. AVM Healthcare. Use of Social Media and Mobile by Healthcare Professionals. 2011; www.amnhealthcare.com/uploadedFiles/AMNHealthcare/Industry-Research/Surveys/final.pdf. Accessed November 7, 2012.

15. Crabtree TD, Puri V, Bell JM, et al. Outcomes and perception of lung surgery with implementation of a patient video education module: a prospective cohort study. *J Am Coll Surg*. 2012;214:816-821. e2. Accessed November 7, 2012.

16. Baum N. How to create YouTube videos for patient education. KevinMD.com. September 2, 2012; www.kevinmd.com/blog/2012/09/create-youtube-videos-patient-education.html. Accessed November 7, 2012.

17. Internet Voice Talent. 30 and 60 Second Spot Word Count Guidelines for Internet Audio Ads. August 6, 2008; www.internetvoicetalent.com/30-and-60-second-spot-word-count-guidelines-for-internet-audio-ads. Accessed November 7, 2012

18. Dugan L. Unofficial Reports Suggest Twitter Surpassed 500M Registered Users In June. AllTwitter blog. July 31, 2012; www.mediabistro.com/alltwitter/twitter-500-million-registered-users_b26104. Accessed November 7, 2012.

19. Twitter Doctors. http://twitterdoctors.net. Accessed November 7, 2012.

20. Chretien KC, Azar J, Kind T. Physicians on Twitter. *JAMA*. 2011;305:566-568.

21. Fox News. CDC Turns to Twitter, Facebook to Promote H1N1 Message. Fox News. 2011; www.foxnews.com/story/0,2933,543962,00.html. Accessed November 7, 2012.

22. Sinclair C. How to use Twitter at your next medical conference. KevinMD.com. September 16, 2011; www.kevinmd.com/blog/2011/09/twitter-medical-conference.html. Accessed November 7, 2012.

23. Blog. Wikipedia, the free encyclopedia. http://en.wikipedia.org/wiki/Blog_(disambiguation). Accessed November 12, 2012.

24. Buzz in the Blogosphere: Millions More Bloggers and Blog Readers. Nielsen Wire. March 8, 2012; http://blog.nielsen.com/nielsenwire/online_mobile/buzz-in-the-blogosphere-millions-more-bloggers-and-blog-readers. Accessed November 12, 2012.

25. Stats. WordPress.com. http://en.wordpress.com/stats. Accessed November 12, 2012.

26. Baerlocher MO, Detsky AS. Online medical blogging: don't do it! *CMAJ*. 2008;179:292.

27. Kovic I, Lulic I, Brumini G. Examining the medical blogosphere: an online survey of medical bloggers. *J Med Internet Res*. 2008;10(3):e28.

28. Manjoo F. How to Blog. Slate. December 18, 2008; www.slate.com/articles/technology/technology/2008/12/how_to_blog.html. Accessed November 12, 2012.

29. Editors. *The Huffington Post Complete Guide to Blogging*. New York: Simon & Schuster; 2008:81.

30. Rowse D. How to Craft Post Titles that Draw Readers Into Your Blog. ProBlogger. August 8, 2008; www.problogger.net/archives/2008/08/20/how-to-craft-post-titles-that-draw-readers-into-your-blog. Accessed November 12, 2012.

31. Gundotra V. Google+. September 17, 2012; https://plus.google.com/+VicGundotra/posts/2YWhK1K3FA5. Accessed December 11, 2012.

> *"If you don't like change, you are going to like irrelevance even less."*
>
> —Eric Shinseki

CHAPTER 5

Rating Sites

INTRODUCTION

Online rating sites—three words that strike fear in the hearts of many doctors. While rating sites are not a new phenomenon, their growth is an evitable outgrowth of broader changes occurring in healthcare. Greater transparency is already evident through the initiatives of leading organizations such as the Centers for Medicare & Medicaid Services (CMS) and Consumer Reports. The patient empowerment goal of the Affordable Care Act will give credibility to patient feedback as an integral part of care. In this day and age, we've become accustomed to rating restaurants, airlines, and other industries online. There is every reason to believe that healthcare will be no exception in a world that increasingly relies on online ratings.

Experts estimate that there are now more than 50 rating sites for healthcare professionals. This chapter details 12 of the leading rating sites. The list was compiled using recent articles in the medical literature and from trending information found on Alexa and Compete, two companies that track Web usage and report metrics. For each rating site profile, information is organized in this manner:

- Scope and demographics: How long the site has been doing doctor ratings and the data it collects and publishes;
- How it works: How consumers can conduct searches for healthcare professionals on the site;
- How providers are rated: The rating system used and any restrictions on use; and
- How providers can interact with the site: How doctors can create their own profiles and manage their account and any other services provided.

The sites profiled here show a range of the type of rating services that are available for patients to use today and the tools that are available for physicians to manage this aspect of their social media presence. While all of them offer somewhat different features, there are many common elements:

- Most use commercially available databases to compile the lists of healthcare professionals on the site. Thus your practice is undoubtedly already listed on most, if not all of these rating sites!

+ Most are free to consumers (exception: Angie's List) and are supported by advertising on the site or by premium services offered to healthcare providers or both.
+ All allow healthcare providers to claim and manage their profile on the site.
+ All offer a search function as well as a rating service, so consumers looking for a doctor can start their search on the site, read what other patients have said, and ultimately provide their own ratings for a given doctor, all on the same site.
+ While exact wording varies, rating assessments generally fall into categories for: ease of getting an appointment, amount of time the provider spent with the patient, wait times, provider's knowledge and bedside manner, staff courtesy, and practice environment.
+ Most sites use a star rating system, along with an option for patients to write narrative comments. A major exception is the new Google+ Local service that uses the Zagat-style rating system of 30 points.

In fact, Google+ Local has the potential to be a game-changer here. Because of its standing as the number 1 search engine and its intent to provide more locally relevant business information, any reviews posted by patients to your Google+ Local listing are likely to be highly visible. When potential patients search on Google, the data to the right of the search results list may include a prominent map and relevant content from your Google+ page, along with reviews.

Where the rating sites differ is in their scope, their approach to handling negative reviews, and the way they interact with healthcare providers:
+ Some sites (e.g., Healthgrades) operate solely in the healthcare industry, while others (e.g., Yelp, Kudzu) are general business sites that have added doctor reviews to their service based on consumer interest. The former may have more reviews, but the latter may have greater visibility and grow in importance as more reviews are posted.
+ Sites vary widely on their guidelines for doctors to follow in responding to reviews and on their response to doctors' requests to have reviews removed.

Information on each of the rating sites presented here was retrieved from two sources: publically available data on the website at the time this book was written and details provided by staff at each rating site in response to our specific questions. Most sites seem genuinely interested in helping doctors maintain a good online profile.

Nevertheless, you may read critical articles, blog posts, and other commentary about the rating sites from doctors who have had bad experiences. One physician, Kent Sepkowitz, MD, undertook his own study of several review sites and wrote about it in a 2008 Slate article. He actually found few posted reviews, which is not surprising in light of the fact that five years ago, this trend hadn't yet really hit healthcare. Sepkowitz's informal study did expose some kinks in the system. He found it to be easy to manipulate, content-poor, and focused on maximizing advertising revenue. He compares the process to that used by eBay, where checks, balances, and reciprocity have led to a robust and reliable rating system.[1]

Other authors have addressed important ethical issues surrounding the use of physician rating sites.[2] Much work remains to be done before physician rating sites can provide the kind of transparency that will positively affect healthcare. The bottom line today is that these sites aren't going away, and doctors should at the very least be familiar with the landscape.

Read how Jamie Cesaretti, MD, a radiation oncologist in Florida, uses rating site profiles to build his new practice:

> When I relocated my radiation oncology practice from Jacksonville to Tampa, Florida, I had to figure out how to compete against urologists in a market that was radically different from the one I had left. Unlike their peers in Jacksonville, Tampa urologists owned their own radiation centers, guaranteeing I wouldn't receive referrals from them.
>
> To break the referral pattern, I updated and posted my physician profile for free on an online physician directory, ratings, and reputation management website. I added new biographical details, contact information, and a link to my website. More importantly, I optimized the profile by including keywords such as "prostrate treatment," "radiation therapy for prostate cancer," "Tampa stereotactic body radiosurgery," and "prostate brachytherapy" to earn good placement in Google searches.
>
> Practically every practice has a website for marketing purposes. But that alone is not enough to attract and retain patients. Individuals now routinely go online to search for the "best doctors" in their city and learn what patients say about their face-to-face experience with those doctors and their employees. That is a major reason I spend around two hours a week checking what is written about me in physician rating sites and asking patients to post reviews online.
>
> I also track and monitor my online reputation to ensure the profiles and ratings prospective patients read about me are accurate. For example, some physician profiling and ratings by insurers could mischaracterize the quality of care I provide because the profiles are based on cost, not quality measures. If that happens, I will know and be ready to explain to patients why I think the rating is unfair.

If a patient writes a negative review, I will respond publicly if the complaint is about my bedside manner, wait time, staff courtesy, or office interior. However, I will handle privately any comments questioning my quality of care and competency to protect patient privacy and avoid getting into a public argument where everybody loses.

If you are not leveraging the many online tools to manage your reputation on the Internet and attract new business to your practice, now is the time to get onboard. Your website is no longer enough.

Jamie Cesaretti, MD
Radiation Oncologist
Winter Park, Florida
www.jamiecesaretti.com

Angie's List

www.angieslist.com

Scope and Demographics

Angie's List (Figure 5.1) started in 1995 as a small company in Columbus, Ohio. The service is now nationwide, although it primarily serves major metropolitan areas. It provides ratings and reviews on a wide variety of service providers—plumbers, contractors, and electricians, for example. Angie's List launched its healthcare service in response to members who were already using Angie's List to find reliable service companies and wanted that same resource to find quality healthcare providers.

Angie's List is the only review site profiled here that charges consumers a membership fee. (The exception is that in some cities where Angie's List is still building lists, it allows customers to use the service for free for the first few months.) Member fees support customer service staff, a monthly magazine, resources such as the *Healthcare Blue Book*, and a complaint-resolution service.

Ratings for physicians/healthcare providers began in March 2008. The site's healthcare activity is up significantly, with searches almost doubling between 2011 and 2012. The number of published reviews is also up significantly. Nationwide, Angie's List receives more than 65,000 new reviews each month in all categories. Although it does not disclose the total number of reviews on the site, Angie's List has reviews for providers in more than 150 specialties in the United States. The service has iPhone, iPad, and Android apps.

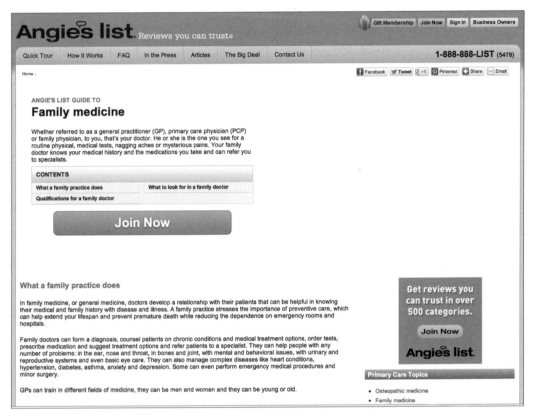

Figure 5.1

Searches generally exceed three million per month, including searches for non-healthcare categories. Angie's List does not automatically include every healthcare provider in its database. A provider is included in the list only after a member submits a report and grades his or her experience.

The typical Angie's List member lives in a two-person household, is between the ages of 35 and 64, owns his or her home, has a college degree, and has an annual household income of at least $100,000.

How It Works

Only members are allowed access to the search function of the site. From the homepage, a consumer can search for a type of provider; the site will use the member's home address (or address used in creating account) as the default. Results can be sorted by distance, grade, reviews, and other factors. For example, searching for "pediatrician–primary care" within 25 miles of 19087, generates 135 results. Of those, 68 have an "A" rating and at least one review, 6 have a "B" rating, and the rest have lower ratings. Clicking on a provider's name brings up a brief profile. Most of the space on the provider page is allocated to reporting patient ratings. All of the graded ratings are shown, followed by full narrative reviews with dates of review.

Staff members at Angie's List believe that consumers are:

" . . . not predisposed to rant about a negative experience. Rather, they're primed to make a connection for some type of treatment, and they're looking for information that will lead them to have a positive experience. When they report on their own experience, it's generally to assign a high grade, which helps perpetuate the cycle of good service/good grades/more business."

How Providers Are Rated

Members can access the review part of the site directly from the homepage, under the tab for "Write a Review," which takes them to a page where they can search for the provider they want to review, or they can go to "Recently Viewed Providers" to begin the review process.

Providers are rated on an A to F scale (A = Excellent; F = Lousy) for eight aspects of care: availability, office environment, punctuality, staff friendliness, bedside manner, communication, effectiveness of treatment, and billing/administration. Consumers are also asked if they would go to this provider again in the future and to provide details of their experience if they wish. Finally, consumers are asked, "How did it go overall?" and encouraged to tell the story of their experience "from start to finish." Responses can be up to 10,000 characters (about 2000 words). Before submitting the review, the consumer will be asked to confirm that the review is true and based on first-hand experience and that he or she is not a competitor to the provider reviewed.

In addition to charging for its services, Angie's List differs from other rating sites in another significant way: it does not allow anonymous postings. This policy can be a double-edged sword for healthcare providers. While it increases the authenticity of individual reports, it may discourage people who would prefer to make their comments anonymously, especially when posting reviews that concern personal health issues. The accountability process at Angie's List also includes proprietary technology, human investigation, and an annual independent audit to determine the validity of reviews.

How Providers Can Interact with Angie's List

As a healthcare provider, you can register at the site to monitor and respond to reviews free of charge. You cannot pay to be added to Angie's List. If your ratings average A or B, you may advertise on the site by giving discounts to members but doing so does not affect the ratings. If your rating falls below a B, this service is no longer allowed.

In creating a profile on the site, you must follow a template but you are encouraged to present as much information about your practice, specialties, accreditations, licensing, and so forth as you want. The service encourages physicians to respond to reviews posted about them. Those who earn and can maintain high grades are also often used as expert sources in the site's magazine and content outlets.

If you contact Angie's List to report a fraudulent review, Angie's List investigators will examine the review, interview the member who submitted it, and investigate to determine appropriate action. The site offers a conflict-resolution service. Angie's List rarely removes reviews because of its accountability process, which it believes tends to discourage attempts to game the system. However, if a report is determined by the site's investigation to be fraudulent, Angie's List will remove it.

Doctor.com

www.doctor.com

Scope and Demographics

Launched in 2008, Doctor.com (Figure 5.2) goes beyond offering tools for consumers to search for and rate doctors by providing premium services empowering providers

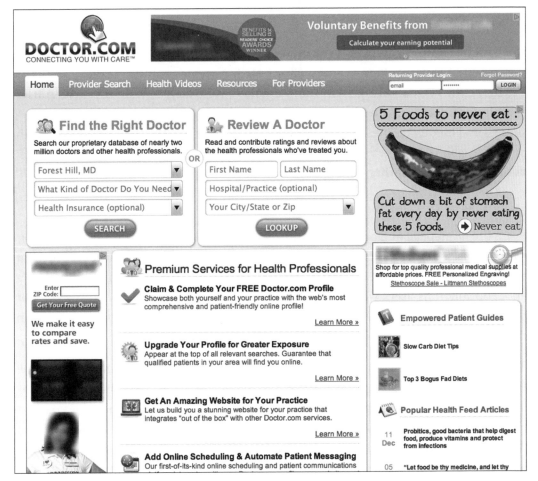

Figure 5.2

to leverage the Web to generate new business and showcase their practice. Those services include helping healthcare professionals establish online credibility, increase awareness of their practice, generate new business, and strengthen relationships with patients.

The site has 2.5 million profiles for most licensed healthcare providers in the United States, including physicians, dentists, nurses, behavioral health professionals, and alternative medicine practitioners. Users can filter their searches by location, specialty, accepted health insurance plans, and other specific criteria. A mobile app is in development.

Doctor.com tracks demographic data on its users and has found that the site is predominantly used by college-educated women aged 35+ with annual income over $80,000. While exact numbers are not available, Doctor.com indicates that "hundreds of thousands of patients" visit the site each month and contribute hundreds of new reviews monthly. It is expanding the number of reviews on the site through partnerships with other sites that have been gathering feedback. Overall, the site has about 20,000 reviews posted.

Doctor.com notes year-over-year increases in the both the total number of new reviews and the percentage of users who contribute reviews. Interestingly, when the site made the review/rating form more detailed, it actually saw an increase in user submissions. Doctor.com also focuses on establishing a community between consumers and medical professionals. Patients can rate and review their experience with providers who've treated them. Healthcare providers can respond to these comments, network with one another, and engage new potential patients through the site.

How It Works

From the homepage of Doctor.com, consumers can search for a healthcare provider, or they can go directly into the review part of the site. The search function on that page, however, is limited to location (zip code or city and state), specialty, and insurance (optional). If users want to do a name search, they go to the tab for "Provider Search," where they are given the same search options as at the homepage or can choose to search under the category "Look up or review a doctor you know."

The site defaults to the zip code of the computer doing the search, so going to the Provider Search page brings up a list of doctors immediately. Searching for a "family doctor" in the 19087 zip code generated eight profiles. None of them had patient ratings, but each had a score called "Doc Points," a measure of the completeness of the provider's profile. The purpose of this rating is to show consumers which profiles have the most information about the doctor's practice; no qualitative assessment is involved in calculating this score. Profiles with the highest scores are listed first.

In the example here, all eight providers had a score of either 20 or 25 (out of 80 possible points), meaning their profiles were missing quite a lot of information. None of the profiles had photos of the doctor, for example. The profile includes basic information of practice address and phone number, specialty, languages spoken, if accepting new patients, education, residency, and board certification. Other aspects such as experience, procedures offered, and affiliated hospitals can be added only by the doctor. If the profile has not been claimed, the site indicates that the information has not been provided.

How Providers Are Rated

A button to "Rate this Provider" is displayed on the profile page. On the review page, patients are first given instructions to read the review guidelines and follow the terms of use. Review guidelines center around three main points: fairness and accuracy; avoiding accusations, insults, and abusive language; and not sharing personally identifiable information.

The ratings page is divided into narrative and star ratings. The patient is asked to provide a short review title, summarizing his or her opinion of the provider. Then space is given for the patient to describe his or her experience with the provider and then assign one overall rating between one and five stars. There are separate star categories for office and staff evaluation—ease of getting appointment, courtesy of office staff, appearance of office, handling of billing/insurance—and a drop-down menu to select wait time. Provider evaluation includes willingness to spend time with the patient, accuracy of diagnosis, and post-visit follow-up.

The patient must give his or her name, but then selects the name as it will appear along with the review: first name, last initial; initials only; or anonymous. The patient must enter a valid e-mail address but that will not be shown on the site; however, a city and state or zip code will be noted in the review.

How Providers Can Interact with Doctor.com

You are encouraged to claim and manage your listing. You have total control over all aspects of your information, and the more complete a profile is, the higher it will rank in search results. In addition, the profile will have a higher Doc Points score and will, therefore be listed higher on Doctor.com searches. By creating an account, you can monitor and respond to reviews and view detailed profile performance reports. Doctor.com also has a mechanism for large multi-location practices to claim and manage profiles for all their individual locations (and the providers who work at them) from within a single account.

Doctor.com has initial filters in place to ensure that any obviously objectionable or defamatory reviews never appear in the first place. No reviews ever appear on the site without being subjected to this filtering. If a provider flags a review and makes a strong case for why it should not be displayed, Doctor.com will typically respond by removing it. The site reserves the right to remove a review at any time for any reason. The site offers support to providers by e-mail, phone, or live chat.

Doctor.com offers several paid premium services for healthcare providers: a syndication service, practice website, and full-service visibility and reputation consultation. The syndication service means that when you update your profile, Doctor.com automatically sends the information to "hundreds of top search and directory sites." This service also allows you to have ads removed from your profile page when it comes up in a patient search. The website option provides for a custom-designed and hosted site for your practice with added features such as online scheduling and social media integration. The reputation consultation option is a full-service marketing plan that is oriented toward optimizing online profiles, defending inaccurate reviews, monitoring reputation, and attracting new patients.

DrScore

www.drscore.com

Scope and Demographics

DrScore (Figure 5.3) is operated by the Medical Quality Enhancement Corp., founded by Steven R. Feldman, MD, PhD. It began its rating service in 2005. DrScore is an interactive online survey site where patients can find as well as rate physicians. More than just a rating site, DrScore uses benchmarks to compare ratings on patient satisfaction and provides detailed survey data to physicians. In addition, the site has a number of articles featuring scientific studies on patient satisfaction. DrScore also partners with patient advocacy groups to help connect patients with advocacy groups and help advocacy groups meet recurring demand for physician information.

DrScore has 800,000 U.S. doctor profiles on the site, providing information on specialty, locations, contact information, and education. All outpatient specialties are represented. Only doctors in the United States are included. If for some reason a doctor is not on the list, consumers can complete a form to request the doctor be added. DrScore will contact the state medical board to verify the information and then add the doctor to the database. In addition to the site, DrScore has an iPhone app called "ineedadoc" that contains the same functionality and content.

The website gets about 300,000 visits per month. Demographic data from the DrScore 2011 Annual Report Card show that two-thirds of patients providing ratings were women and that a broad patient age range is represented in the ratings, with over

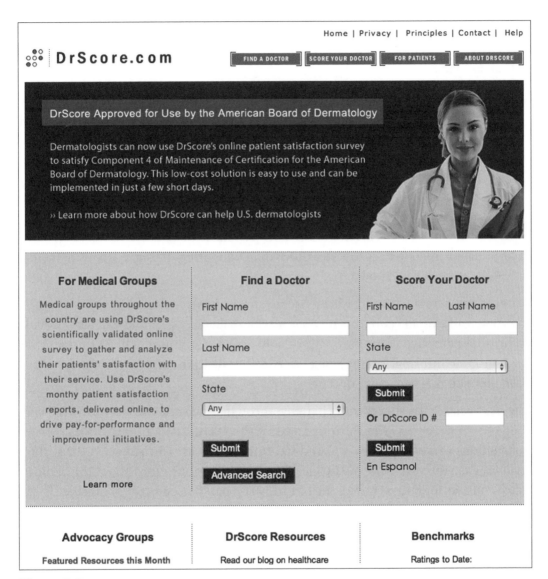

Figure 5.3

1600 children and 500 adults over the age of 65. As of October 2012, there are over 250,000 ratings on DrScore. Ratings are growing at a rapid pace. In 2011, the site got about 3000 posted each month; and as of late 2012, that number had risen to 4500 per month, a 50% increase.

How It Works

To find a physician, consumers need to search using at least the doctor's last name and state. The search engine will alert the user when it needs additional information. For example, if someone searches without putting in a last name, the results page may indicate that more than 250 physicians were found. In that case, the search engine would ask the consumer to provide more information. When patients ask for information about doctors in a particular medical specialty, DrScore not only provides that information, but also information about patient advocacy groups related to that specialty.

When patients go to DrScore in search of a doctor, only five ratings are shown: an overall rating (scale of 1 to 10), along with the number of ratings and the date of the most recent rating, and overall ratings for Exam, Timeliness, Treatment, and Staff.

How Providers Are Rated

Patients can rate their physicians anonymously on DrScore. Patients are limited to rating each doctor only once per quarter to prevent them from skewing the ratings by repeatedly rating a doctor in a short time period. The site has internal controls to determine if someone tries to enter more than one rating. If that action is detected, only one rating will be shown.

Patients can rate doctors in a brief online survey in six steps. They are first asked to provide an overall score for the doctor on a scale of 1 to 10 and can also provide additional narrative comments, up to a 40-word maximum. They are asked for demographic information (age, sex, race, and education) and how long they have been going to this particular doctor.

The next page of the survey takes patients through nine variables regarding the care they received, such as the thoroughness of the exam, the amount of time spent, instructions received, follow-up, and treatment success. The same 1 to 10 scale is used for each question. The next page of the survey has questions about the clinic or office and asks for ratings (on a scale of 1 to 10) on parking, courtesy of office staff, etc.

A separate section of the survey asks patients how many days it took to get an appointment with the doctor, how many minutes they waited in the office before seeing the doctor, and how many minutes the doctor spent with them. Finally, patients are asked to identify any area in which they believe the doctor's practice could have been better (e.g., office staff, getting appointments, getting information over the telephone).

Scores are generally high on DrScore. In its 2011 Annual Report, the site reported that of the 298 doctors with 10 ratings or more, the mean score was 9.2; 62% of ratings were a perfect 10. For all 36,000 ratings in the database, average scores increased from 7.07 in 2010 to 7.12 in 2011. Scores for primary care doctors and specialists were about equal. DrScore also has functionality for patients to provide narrative comments, but those reviews are not displayed on the website. The information is, however, provided to doctors who use the DrScore patient satisfaction feedback service.

How Providers Can Interact with DrScore

You can set up your own profile on DrScore. As long as you remain in practice, the site will carry a listing; the basic profile cannot be removed upon request. You can also purchase the more detailed information collected by the ratings survey. DrScore reports can be accessed through the site's online reporting system. The reports include your mean scores and scores for the office practice and the staff, each with a comparison to benchmark data on U.S. physicians and physicians in the same specialty. Patients' open comments are also included. The DrScore report describes in detail potential problem areas pointed out by patients.

The DrScore survey has been recognized as valid by the U.S. Agency for Healthcare Research and Quality, and its data have been used in peer-reviewed medical publications. DrScore gives you the ability to collect surveys for your practice.

DrScore believes that fraudulent reviews are not a major issue on its site because it posts only mean numerical ratings, not narrative reviews. If you believe a rating is unfair or unrepresentative of your practice, DrScore believes the best solution is for you to encourage more of your patients to do ratings. This process would allow you to correct misrepresentations and, more importantly, find out if there really is a problem in the practice that can be corrected or improved.

Google+ Local

www.google.com/+/learnmore/local

Scope and Demographics

We know from research studies conducted by Pew that 72% of Internet users search online for health information.[3] That number is more telling than the total number of Google+ users because as a search engine, Google has the ability to reach anyone, anywhere who is looking for information on a healthcare provider. Increasingly, the search result will not only lead to a website or to rating sites, but to a prominent Google+ Local listing of the medical practice, along with prominently placed reviews. Now the world's most popular search engine is also potentially the most visible rating site.

Google+ Local (Figure 5.4) was created by merging Google Places with Google Maps. It was launched May 30, 2012, by automatically converting 80 million Google Places pages to Google+ Local pages. This conversion occurred even if a business had not claimed its Google Places profile. If Google has a map of your practice, chances are you are already listed in Google+ Local.

How It Works

Consumers can find Google+ Local pages through a Google.com search, on a search of Google Maps, or directly through Google+, on the Web or through mobile apps. Google+ Local pages can appear in search results for general categories (e.g.,

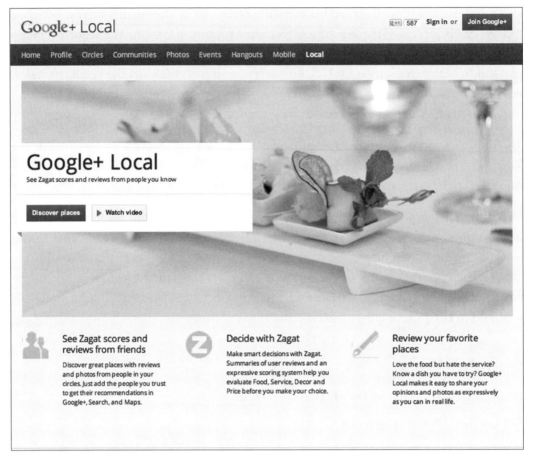

Figure 5.4

"pediatrician" + zip code) or in a Google search for a specific doctor. For example, a general search for "pediatrician, 19087" generated a Google map showing seven local practices (labeled A to G on the map) with corresponding links to the Google+ page of each physician. A search in Google Maps generated a few more listings (A to J) with associated links. A name search would show similar results.

Clicking on the link for "plus.google.com" below any doctor's name in the search results brings up the profile page. It includes a large map, address, phone number, and any photos or additional information provided by the doctor. Reviews posted through Google+ are also included, as are links to reviews on other websites, such as Citysearch or Vitals.

How Providers Are Rated

From the page of any business, including medical practices, consumers can click "Write a review." Google has done away with its previous star rating system in favor of the rating system popularized by Zagat, which uses scores and summaries compiled from user reviews. There are no anonymous reviews on Google+ Local. All reviews appear under the user's name and are displayed to anyone who views that person's profile on Google+, anyone who searches for places if they've added you to their Google+ circles, and anyone who views places you've reviewed. All scores in Google+ Local are determined by user reviews.

The unique scoring system uses 30 points and ranges from "poor" to "perfection." While most people associate these ratings with food, service, and décor in Zagat's restaurant guides, Google is now using the system for all of its Google+ Local business reviews. The summaries highlight quotes from real users to help consumers make informed decisions.

Individual user ratings work on a scale of 0 to 3, with 3 being excellent and 0 being poor to fair. Google then averages the ratings, multiplying by 10 to arrive at an average score on a 30-point scale. Total scores fall into the following categories:

- 26–30: Extraordinary to perfection
- 21–25: Very good to excellent
- 16–20: Good to very good
- 11–15: Fair to good
- 0–10: Poor to fair

How Providers Can Interact with Google+ Local

First, claim your listing. Google+ accounts are designed for individuals, not businesses or medical practices. Information regarding practice details belongs on Google+ Local so that it can be paired with the map functionality Google uses in its local listings. Go to http://plus.google.com/pages/create. Chances are, your practice will already appear on a search results page, along with a map and a link to Google+. You may have already noticed changes if you had a Google Place page—it has been or soon will be automatically converted into a Google+ Local page.

It's important to claim your listing because users will now be able to find your page through a Web or map search on Google, through a mobile app, or from a search directly on Google+. Search results showing your practice along with a map are more visually appealing and thus more likely to get click-throughs from potential patients.

Google+ Local listings are compiled from online directories. As a result, your practice likely already exists as a Google+ Local page. You can find it in several ways. First, if you want to check out the competition, you can do a general search for doctors in your area (e.g., "internal medicine, Nashua, NH"). Your name will probably appear on a list with similar doctors and a map noting the location of each. Find a link to your Google+ page beneath your name in the search results, where you can select

"Manage this page." You will then be taken to the homepage for Google Places for Business where you can sign in and begin editing your business information.

In addition to address, phone number, website, and description, you can list your hours of operation and post photos or videos. When you have completed your profile, hit the "Submit" button. Google has a verification process for Google+ Local pages that are created. After you complete your page listing, Google will ask you to confirm your address and will mail you a postcard via snail mail so you can confirm that you updated your business listing.

You can also claim your business listing by a search using your business telephone number. Fill in basic information, such as your practice address, website, and a short description of the practice.

Finally, add links on your website to the Google+ Local page.

Google has procedures for removing reviews. A business owner can flag a review as inappropriate to report it. Google will check to see if the review violates any of its stated guidelines such as unlawful content, spam, off-topic review, or conflict of interest. However, Google cautions businesses that "more often than not, we leave the review up."

Healthcare Reviews

www.healthcarereviews.com

Scope and Demographics

Healthcare Reviews (Figure 5.5) began rating doctors and other healthcare professionals in July 2006. The site has over 1.4 million profiles of doctors, dentists, and other healthcare professionals in 33 specialties. The practitioners are primarily in the United States; fewer than 100,000 are Canadian and international.

The company does not track the demographics of its users and has not produced any reports on usage statistics. The number of ratings on its site is not publically available.

How It Works

Users are given two choices when they enter the site: either "Search Ratings" or "Submit Reviews." Searches can be done in four categories: doctors, dentists, hospitals and clinics, and all healthcare professionals. If a patient selects the search function and looks for all practitioners in a given location and specialty (without searching by name), the results will be capped at 100 listings. Searches can be refined by adding a provider's last name or partial last name. Rated doctors are listed first, but there might be only a few listings. Many results will be of unrated doctors.

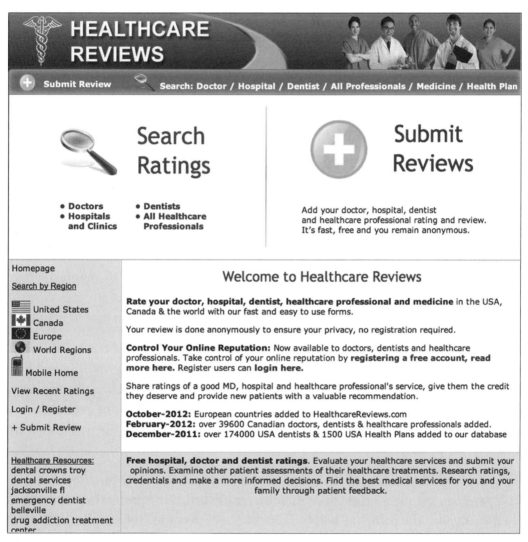

Figure 5.5

Clicking on a doctor's name brings up a profile with location and contact information, followed by ratings. Although Healthcare Reviews does not have an app, it does have a mobile site available for use with smartphones at www.healthcarereviews.com/m.

How Providers Are Rated

By selecting "Submit Reviews," users are taken through a three-step process. After selecting a category and state, they go to a page to enter the healthcare professional's name. The provider's sex and specialty must also be provided to continue. If the system recognizes the name entered, the next page will ask users to confirm that this is the person they are seeking to review. The users are then asked to give an overall rating on a scale of 1 to 10 (where 10 is "very good," 5 is "ok," and 1 is "poor"). Users can also provide optional ratings in these areas:

- Wait Times (10 = quick; 1 = long waits);
- Helpful (10 = very helpful; 1 = rude);
- Knowledgeable (10 = intelligent; 1 = overconfident); and
- Cost/fees: (10 = good deal; 1 = too expensive).

Users can submit brief narrative comments of up to 250 characters that will be displayed in a separate section of the provider's profile below the numerical ratings.

How Providers Can Interact with Healthcare Reviews

Healthcare Reviews' goal is to work with physicians, hospitals, and healthcare professionals to provide ratings and reviews that they value and to provide a free account for professionals to use to manage their online reputation and interact with patients. When you register with the site, you can interact with patients by replying to their comments and can even remove comments deemed slanderous or inappropriate. You can also choose to receive e-mail alerts of patient comments and can control what contact information is displayed when your name appears in search results.

If your rating already exists in the database, you can contact Healthcare Reviews with your registration details and the Web page of the current listing; the site will link your registration details to the existing rating. You can edit all publically displayed information at any time. The site gives you control over your online reputation. If you respond to posted patient reviews, the replies are publically displayed directly beneath the patient comments.

Hospitals and clinics can list their members by contacting Healthcare Reviews. The company can list all members in its directory, rather than the hospital staff having to do it manually. The company will then register free accounts for hospital and clinic professional staff members to better control their online reputation. Healthcare Reviews can also help provide custom ratings and feedback reports for an organization's internal needs on a contractual basis.

Healthgrades

www.healthgrades.com

Scope and Demographics

Healthgrades (Figure 5.6) began providing objective measures of hospital performance in 1998 and introduced physician quality information in 2000. In 2004, Healthgrades introduced an instrument to measure patient satisfaction consistently and objectively. Rather than subjective open comments, its patient satisfaction surveys feature seven questions representing the measures that patients are most likely to use to recommend a doctor. (See How Providers Are Rated for specific measures.)

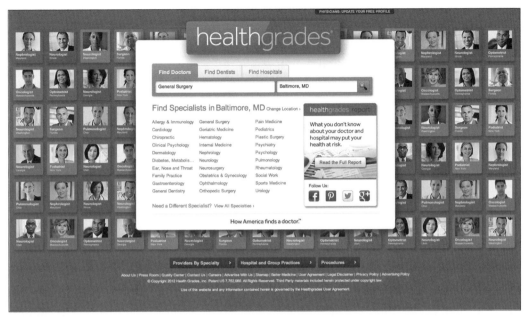

Figure 5.6

Every physician licensed to practice in the United States is featured on Healthgrades, with content licensed and collected from public and private sources. Healthgrades includes profiles of about one million physicians in more than 100 specialties and more than five million profiles of other healthcare professionals (i.e., dentists, mental health professionals, chiropractors, nurse practitioners, physician assistants), 5000 hospitals, and 16,000 nursing homes. It is solely a U.S. company. As a robust source of data, Healthgrades appears on the first page of a Google search of a provider's name 99% of the time. The Healthgrades profile is among the top three Google listings 95% of the time.

More than 200 million people use Healthgrades annually to find, select, and connect with healthcare professionals. Usage statistics show 77% of them plan to visit a physician within 30 days. In addition, 74% of people searching Healthgrades consider two or more physicians for the current medical issue before making an appointment. Healthgrades analyzes site visitor demographics and finds that 73% of visitors to the site are commercially insured, 72% are female, 84% have at least a secondary education, and 52% have annual household income over $75,000.

By the end of 2012, it expects to have received three million patient surveys, across nearly 655,000 providers, which Healthgrades believes is the largest collection in the industry. Healthgrades enables patients to search and evaluate providers on the website, partner sites, and a mobile site (launched in June 2012).

How It Works

From the homepage, users enter the specialty they are seeking or a provider's name, then the area (by zip code) where they are seeking information. A search quickly produces a list of potential doctors. For example, a search for "internal medicine" and "Villanova, PA," produced a list of 950 potential doctors within 10 miles.

Users can narrow the search by distance (as few as five miles), provider's sex, type of insurance accepted by the practice, and quality variables (including patient recommendations). To continue with this example, if the search is restricted to doctors within five miles of Villanova *and* those recommended by patients, the list is narrowed to 53 names. Nearly all physicians in the list were recommended by 100% of patients who reviewed them on the site. Results such as these are consistent with data suggesting that most online reviews of physicians are positive.

Clicking on a specific physician's listing will bring up a page with tabs for basic information such as age and education, office locations, appointment information and maps, and the results of background checks and patient satisfaction surveys.

Healthgrades believes consumer decision-making is based on a set of key objective measures, and that a patient's choice of physician is inextricably linked to his or her choice of hospital. Thus hospital affiliations and quality scores are included in every profile.

How Providers Are Rated

Healthgrades' physician profiles differentiate doctors across five key attributes: personal, practice, professional, procedural, and performance criteria. Its Patient Satisfaction Survey includes ratings for both the patient's experience in the office (scheduling appointments, office environment and friendliness, wait time) as well as with the provider (level of trust, helps patient understand his or her condition, listen/answers questions, and time spent with patient.) Patients can simply go to the physician's profile page and click on "Take the Survey."

Healthgrades also compiles outcomes data from dozens of independent public and private sources including CMS, 19 states' records of all payer data, 50 states' medical board records, and publicly available directories. That information is summarized in a background report with each provider's profile. Physician data are updated quarterly.

Healthgrades has a rigorous process for electronic validation of every patient satisfaction survey submitted, and it restricts the number of surveys a patient can complete on a physician.

How Providers Can Interact with Healthgrades

In 2011, Healthgrades launched a Physician and Provider Portal for healthcare providers to update their own profile information. The portal, which is a free and secure online application, also provides physicians with customized profile activity reports and other useful tools. Healthgrades' research has shown that patients are most interested in finding information on the five areas listed below:

- Insurance accepted;
- Photo and video;
- Care philosophy;
- Conditions treated; and
- Procedures performed.

Thus the new portal encourages you to address all of these aspects of your practice and to keep your profile updated to ensure accuracy. In fact, Healthgrades claims that patients are more than twice as likely to engage with physicians who have a complete profile than with those who use only the standard profile. You simply need to register on the site to take advantage of this application. You and your practice managers have control over the profile, with the ability to enhance, edit, and update more than 75 professional and practice details that help patients choose a provider.

In addition to the profile, Healthgrades offers several tools that are specifically designed to help manage your online reputation. You can track profile visits and patient satisfaction survey activity and compare results with other providers. You can also respond to patient surveys by posting a public response. The portal contains patient satisfaction surveys that can be printed to hand out or mail to patients. Getting more survey results helps build credible scores and attract more patients.

Healthgrades' procedures designed to prevent patient survey fraud, as described above, limit the number of contested ratings. But if you feel that a false survey has been posted, you are invited to contact Healthgrades to investigate the matter to ensure the reliability of the source of the review. Healthgrades will not add surveys that have not been validated. And after an investigation into a potentially fraudulent survey has been completed, it will remove a survey that is found to be falsely submitted.

Insider Pages

www.insiderpages.com/doctorfinder

Scope and Demographics

Insider Pages was created to help people find local businesses through recommendations from their friends and neighbors. On the site, people share reviews of local businesses such as restaurants and hair salons, to find services they can trust. Launched

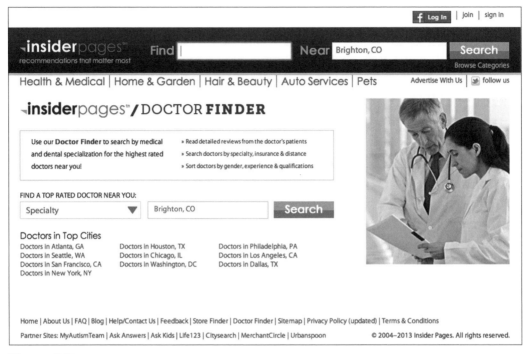

Figure 5.7

in 2004, Insider Pages is headquartered in the San Francisco Bay area. It was acquired by Citysearch, a local search, directory, and media company that is part of IAC, in March 2007, but remains a separate brand.

In May 2010, Insider Pages launched Doctor Finder (Figure 5.7). The site covers about one million doctors and other healthcare professionals in the United States, with data from Healthgrades. Physicians, dentists, alternative health practitioners, and many other types of healthcare professionals (e.g., audiologists, physical therapists, nutritionists) are included in Doctor Finder. The site does not publish demographic data, but its Wikipedia entry indicates that "as part of IAC, Insider Pages has grown significantly and now has more than 1.5 million user generated reviews and receives over five million unique visitors each month."[4]

How It Works

Consumers can go to the section of the Insider Pages site for Doctor Finder to begin a search by location and specialty. For example, searching for "cardiologist" in "St. Louis, MO" generated 300 results. The search can then be filtered by insurance accepted and the provider's sex, location, ratings, and years of experience. Refining the above search to female cardiologists with at least 10 years' experience and within five miles of the city produced 14 results. Only one provider had reviews; she was listed first.

The profile includes basic information about the doctor's practice and a summary of ratings (if any). Insider Pages obtains some of its healthcare provider information from Healthgrades, which, in turn, has obtained it from commercial database sources. Insider Pages carries a disclaimer on profiles that have come from Healthgrades that it does not make any representations or warranties on the accuracy or timeliness of its information.

In addition to information about the provider selected, the profile page also contains links to two other nearby doctors.

How Providers Are Rated

From a doctor's profile page, patients can click on "Write a Review" to begin, but they must have an account on Insider Pages to do so. To sign up for an account, a consumer needs to give his or her first name, last initial, zip code, and e-mail address (for confirmation of the account). Patient reviews are based on a 10-question survey. Commonly asked questions are included, such as time spent with the doctor, ease of scheduling the appointment, and courtesy of the office staff. This site also asks patients if they believe the doctor understood their medical condition, listened and answered their questions, and gave trustworthy recommendations. The survey also asks patients to disclose the condition for which they sought care and the treatment they received.

A narrative review must be included, which can be as few as 25 characters or as many as 5000. In addition to the narrative review, users must give one overall rating and a title to their review, but they are not required to answer the entire survey in order to post their review.

According to a published interview with general manager Eric Peacock in 2010, Insider Pages doesn't edit patient reviews, but it also does not allow patients to claim misconduct or malpractice in their reviews.[5]

How Providers Can Interact with Insider Pages

To get started, you must sign up for an account with Insider Pages. Once your account is set up, do a search for your business on the site. When you find your profile page, click the "Claim Business" link for your business listing. You can return to the site and update the information at any time. Click "View/Update Business Profile" for the business you wish to edit.

On this page, you can update your business information, add or change your business categories to include more keywords, provide more information about your expertise, add photos, update types of insurance accepted, and respond to reviews left on your business profile.

You can attempt to have a review removed from your business listing by submitting it to Insider Pages for review. To report a review, sign into your account, go to the review in question, and click "Report Abuse." The site will assess the review to determine if it violates terms and conditions such as containing profanity, allegations of illegal activity, reviews written by current or former employees, and the like. If it violates the terms and conditions, it will be removed. If the review does not violate these terms, it will remain on the site. Insider Pages will notify you of its decision by e-mail. Negative reviews determined to be factual and legitimate will remain on the site.

Kudzu

www.kudzu.com

Scope and Demographics

Kudzu (Figure 5.8) provides free, open-access reviews on home and family services. The name "Kudzu" was chosen because the founders liked the idea of something

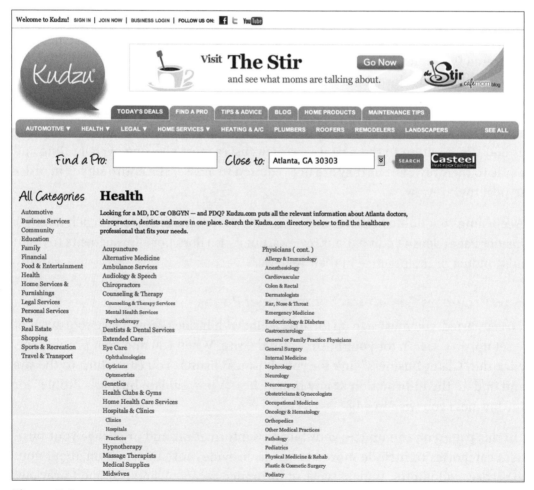

Figure 5.8

fast-growing—like the kudzu vine—and felt that good word of mouth spreads quickly. Launched in 2006, Kudzu features more than four million consumer reviews and detailed business profiles built by local service providers. The company is a division of Cox Enterprises, a large media company based in Atlanta, Georgia. The initial focus was on home services, but since 2011, Kudzu has placed increased emphasis on additional categories including doctors and healthcare and financial and legal services.

Kudzu has more than 1.5 million unique visitors per month, with approximately 14% searching for doctors. More than 15,000 new reviews are posted each month. As of September 2012, there were 66,086 healthcare reviews on Kudzu. The site has seen an increase in reviews posted in the past 12 months of 10% to 45%, depending on the category. A recent internal survey indicates that 94% of registered Kudzu users look at reviews prior to going to a healthcare provider.

Kudzu attracts a targeted, affluent audience. Its customer base is 93% homeowners with a median household income of $93,000. The majority are married and female, with 72% between the ages of 25 and 54. Kudzu has a large, engaged user base and plans to make ongoing investments to further grow the healthcare category.

Kudzu has more than 162,000 health profiles on the site, and the number is growing. Specialties include most areas of clinical medicine and other categories such as hospitals and clinics, and weight management centers. Currently only U.S. doctors are listed.

How It Works

Consumers can begin searches by entering a location and the type of professional they are looking for. The top of the search results page includes several ads for providers or other services in the same geographic area. Search results can then be sorted by distance, rankings, and other variables. A random look at cardiologists in Atlanta showed that of 379 listed, only 50 actually had reviews associated with their profile. Clicking on a search result brings up a profile with three tabs: "Overview," "Map," and "Reviews." A section called "Top-Rated" appears at the top and features doctors who have top five ratings. The Reviews tab includes "What your neighbors are saying" for the reviews that Kudzu users have posted; and if there are no Kudzu-original reviews, a heading of "Reviews from around the web" may appear with reviews from other sites such as Citysearch.

Registered users of Kudzu can save custom search settings for faster searches. Recent searches are automatically saved so that they are easier to retrieve. Users are encouraged to complete a profile. In February 2009, Kudzu joined with Facebook Connect to allow consumers to sign in with their Facebook ID and share reviews with friends. In May 2009, Kudzu connected with Twitter to allow users to share their favorites.

Kudzu also offers iPhone and Android apps that enable consumers to conduct location-based searches and view detailed business profiles with phone numbers, maps, and directions, plus customer reviews, photos, and special offers to help choose the best service provider while on the go.

How Providers Are Rated

Only registered users can publish reviews on Kudzu. To protect the credibility of reviews, it allows consumers to review a business only once. When users click on "Write Review" on any professional's profile page, they are encouraged to write about their first-hand experiences and include the kinds of information they'd want to get when asking a friend about a business. Users are encouraged to review businesses they've been to recently, and to not get personal, use profanity, or claim that businesses broke the law. Kudzu will remove posts that do not follow these guidelines.

Users are also urged to "make it kind" with tips such as this: "Have service pros you would not recommend? Let's not skewer them folks. Just let your neighbors know how your experience did not meet your expectations." Sample positive reviews are included with the writing tips.

The review process involves three steps: In Step 1, users are asked to rate the provider on a one- to five-star scale, on each of four variables: overall, quality, service, and value. The total overall star rating of the reviews is rounded to the nearest half star. In Step 2, users are asked to give a title to their review. Step 3 provides space for a narrative review of up to 250 words. Reviews posted on Kudzu must comply with the site's Visitor Agreement that stipulates, among other restrictions, that the user will not post any libelous or harmful content.

How Providers Can Interact with Kudzu

Check to see if your practice is already listed on Kudzu. You can search by your business name or by keyword using the search box at the top of any Kudzu page. If you locate your business in the search results, click on the name to see your business profile. On the right side of the profile page, look for the blue box marked "Is this your business?," then click "Register your company today." If your practice is not already published, click the "Got a business? Get it listed" link in the far right column of Kudzu's homepage. You will be taken to a page where you can register your practice, add content, and make corrections.

You can set up a basic profile yourself, and the Kudzu account team can assist with the details for enhanced profile listings. A basic profile includes key contact information, website link, specialties and services, hours of operation, and special offers (if any).

Enhanced profiles enable you to showcase the most important features of your practice, including a detailed description, contact info, logo or other graphics, photos, videos, and any special offers. To ensure highest placement in search engine results, Kudzu advises that healthcare professional upgrade to an enhanced profile.

Kudzu offers a business center that enables you to update your profile information at any time. You can also view reports with key metrics including impressions served (ads displayed to a user), clicks, phone calls, e-mail inquiries, map views, video views, review views, and number of consumers who saved your profile as a favorite.

You have complete control over how your practice information is displayed.

You can also comment on posted reviews. Reviews are overwhelmingly positive—76% of Kudzu users write reviews to express satisfaction. If you believe a review violates the agreement, you can notify the site operations manager who will investigate and remove any noncompliant reviews.

RateMDs

www.ratemds.com

Scope and Demographics

RateMDs (Figure 5.9) was founded in 2004 by John Swapceinski, who also founded RateMyProfessors.com and RateMyTeachers.com. RateMDs receives about two million visits per month, with traffic doubling every year. The site includes over 1.8 million reviews of over 300,000 doctors in the United States, Canada, United Kingdom/Ireland, Australia/New Zealand, India, and South Africa.

RateMDs does not publish any demographic data, but some information can be gleaned from the literature and from Web-tracking sites. In a recent article in the

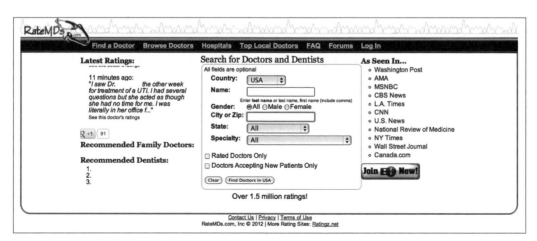

Figure 5.9

Canadian Medical Association Journal, Swapceinski explained that up to 40% of the site's users are from Canada.[6] Canadian doctors are also well-represented—about 90% have at least one rating, as compared with 20% of U.S. doctors. Recent statistics on Alexa, the Web metrics site, indicates that RateMDs gets 54.5% of its traffic from the United States, 30.8% from Canada, 5.5% from India, and 2.4% from Germany. Tracking site Quantcast.com shows that an estimated 460,000 people visited RateMDs each month between January 30 and July 30, 2012. Other demographic data tracked by Quantcast indicate that users are more likely to be older, have no children, have annual incomes in excess of $150,000, and be more educated than the average Internet user.

How It Works

The site is free for consumers to use and is supported by advertising. From the homepage, users can go to "Find a Doctor" and search by either name or location and specialty. (There is also an option to browse doctors by state in the United States or by international location.) Users searching for a particular doctor who is not yet listed in RateMDs have the option of adding the doctor to the site. A search for "family/GP" in "Wayne, PA" filtered to include only those doctors with ratings and accepting new patients generated more than 90 results.

Clicking on the physician's name will bring up a brief profile with the provider's sex, educational background, specialty, practice name, website, and phone number. Other optional information includes a place for the physician to indicate willingness to communicate by e-mail, availability of online scheduling, and if he or she is accepting new patients.

RateMDs relies on visitors to its site to add physicians to the site's listings. A summary of the ratings and number of ratings are included in the basic listing, followed by detailed reviews, including dates.

The site also has some unique compilations such as a list of the top 10 doctors in each specialty for many locations. This list is based on a weighting of the doctor's average overall rating score, along with the number of ratings received. Therefore, a doctor with a somewhat lower average score and many ratings may be listed higher than a doctor with a higher average score and fewer ratings.

In addition to highlighting the best-rated doctors, the site also includes a "Wall of Shame." This list includes doctors who make prospective patients sign "gag contracts" before they are accepted as patients. RateMDs allows users to add to this list by responding to a thread on its forum.

How Providers Are Rated

Ratings are based on a five-point scale and cover four categories—staff, punctuality, helpfulness, and knowledge. The overall quality rating is the average score of the ratings for helpfulness and knowledge. Ratings in the punctual category are not used in computing the overall quality rating for the physician. The overall rating is shown as a numerical average (e.g., 4.3) and a colored "smiley face" representing the nature of the rating as high average, fair average, or low average. Patients can also write narrative reviews of up to 1000 characters but are not required to do so in order to post ratings. Before posting, patients are asked to certify that the rating is based on their own experience with the doctor. However, RateMDs cautions users that this aspect of the service cannot be verified. Thus it encourages users to "take the ratings with a grain of salt."

Comments posted on RateMDs are reviewed; the site reserves the right to delete comments or an entire rating if it is deemed inappropriate. The site also allows consumers to delete a rating as long as the rater can be verified (by signing into an account, for example).

RateMDs uses a spam filter to try to prevent anyone from stuffing the ballot box. If two or more ratings for the same doctor come from the same computer or rater, they are deleted, and a message is posted advising viewers that such duplication has occurred. Thus if you encourage your patients to submit ratings on RateMDs, you should ask that they do so from their home computers and not make this service available from your office computer.

How Providers Can Interact with RateMDs

You cannot submit or maintain a profile for this site. Only consumers can add doctors to the site and post ratings. Furthermore, if your profile is on the site, you cannot have it taken down. However, there is a link to correct any misinformation in the basic listing. You can also respond to reviews by creating a free account on the site. In addition, each rating posted has a red flag beside it. If you have found a rating that you think is libelous or erroneous, you can click on that flag and have the rating sent back to RateMDs' staff to review again along with the reason you want this rating deleted.

RateMDs encourages you to tell patients about its site. Indeed, a study showed that most of its reviews are favorable. Recall the study by Gao et al, mentioned earlier in this book which found that, on average, physicians received a total rating of 3.93 out of 5, with almost 50% getting a perfect 5 rating on RateMDs. The average number of ratings per physician was 3.2 in January 2010.[7]

RateMDs also encourages you to post links to the site from your own practice site. You may also be able to display your RateMDs ratings on your website. Simply go to your ratings page and click on the link "Docs, add these ratings to your website." Only ratings with at least a 4 out of 5 in every category will be displayed.

RateMDs cautions doctors not to rate themselves as a way of getting good reviews online. It warns doctors that this practice, known as "astroturfing," is illegal and has been successfully challenged in court. It cites a case where a cosmetic surgery practice posted a number of false reviews and paid $300,000 to settle the case.

Vitals

www.vitals.com

Scope and Demographics

Vitals (Figure 5.10) is a combination physician and dentist directory and review site. Launched in January 2008, it provides a searchable database of more than 870,000 physicians in the United States, Guam, and Puerto Rico, in more than 200 specialties. Vitals is used by more than nine million people each month; more than 100 million consumers visit Vitals each year. About 50,000 reviews are posted by patients each month on Vitals; the site has more than two million total patient ratings and reviews.

Vitals tracks key information about consumers who use the site. For instance, 85% of patients who visit Vitals see a doctor or visit a hospital within 30 days of doing a Vitals search, and 82% purchased a prescription in the last 30 days for themselves or someone else. Demographic data include 65% of Vitals users are female, 71% are over age 35, 56% have an annual household income in excess of $60,000, and 66% have a college degree.

A recently introduced iPhone app allows users to find and create top-10 lists of the best local doctors, as rated by patients anywhere in the United States. The app also stores information such as doctors' phone numbers and photos of health insurance cards for easy access.

How It Works

Information on Vitals is available to consumers free of charge. Its revenue comes from customized tools and services that Vitals offers to hospitals, health plans, and websites, and from advertising on the site. Consumers can search for a doctor by name, location, specialty, or condition. An interactive graphic feature also allows searching by symptoms if the patient does not know what specialist to see. For example, a search for an allergist within 10 miles of Wilmington, Delaware, identified seven doctors. The user can refine the search further to find a doctor who is board-certified, was educated in the United States, has a three-star rating or higher, or speaks certain languages. The search can also be limited by provider's sex and type of degree (i.e., MD vs. DO). Continuing with the search above, limiting the search to board-certified allergists within 10 miles of Wilmington returned three possibilities.

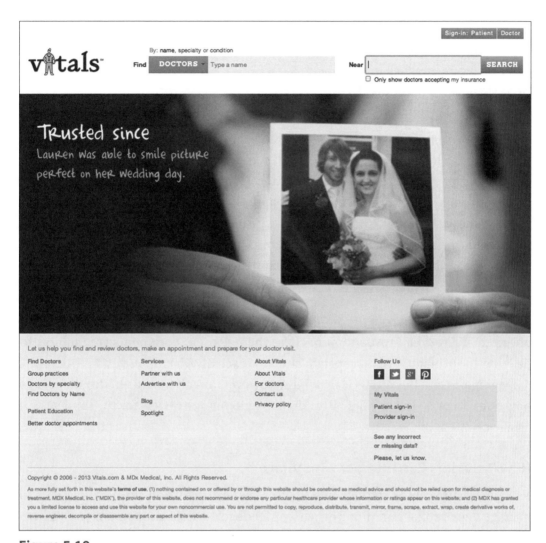

Figure 5.10

Each physician profile includes the practice address and overall patient rating along with specialty information, board certification, hospital affiliations, education, and insurance accepted. The site also has a number of Patient Guides to help patients better prepare for tests and appointments.

Vitals aggregates physician data from a number of sources, including state boards of medicine, hospital websites, publication databases, and award sites (e.g., Top Doctors). Vitals calls it the "360-degree view"—factual information on a doctor's expertise coupled with consumer reviews and recommendations from other doctors. Each doctor's rating is generated by considering four important points of view. The first is reviews obtained by peers and awards given by professional boards. In the second place, the rating for each doctor is formed by patient reviews. The third aspect considered for making a doctor's rating is the factual information, which takes into account expertise and academic background. Lastly, the office information available is also taken into account.

How Providers Are Rated

All patient ratings are based on a scale of one to four stars. The Overall Patient Rating is an average of all responses to the question: "Overall, what is your opinion of this doctor?" The national average overall score is 2.9. Then summary ratings, also on a scale of one to four stars, are shown for each of these criteria: ease of scheduling an appointment, promptness, courteous staff, accurate diagnosis, bedside manner, spends time with patient, and follow-up. The ratings included in the individual doctor's profile are also averages of total responses to each question. Finally, wait times are averaged from all patients who review, and the average is listed and benchmarked against national averages.

Vitals also includes narrative comments from patients. These comments are posted unedited; doctors can respond publicly to them. Patient comments are "subject to deletion for profanity, inappropriate content, excessive harshness and reputation-damaging prose." The numerical ratings, however, are all included. The site allows only one reviewer from a single IP address to submit one review for the same physician every 30 days.

How Providers Can Interact with Vitals

As a physician licensed in the United States, you can create an account on Vitals to manage your profile and monitor patient feedback. Vitals encourages you to help consumers with their choices by ensuring that your profile is complete and accurate. You can add a photograph and update the information in your Vitals profile. Vitals wants you to brag. You are urged to add awards, appointments, and recognitions to your profile.

You can then use your personal Physician Dashboard to monitor your reputation on Vitals. You can review patient comments and share feedback on what they say. In addition, you can edit certain aspects of your profile to ensure it fully reflects you. The site also allows you to publicly respond to consumer comments.

Vitals urges you to be proactive in seeking positive reviews. It provides free, customizable comment cards that can be distributed to patients. The cards contain the basic message "If you're satisfied, tell others on Vitals. If you're not, tell us." Vitals also has a devoted Physician Relations team that investigates suspicious comments and responds to physician concerns.

Finally, Vitals offers several different styles of badges that can be displayed on your practice website to get more reviews and increase visibility, sponsored-link advertising, and press releases to promote achievements and awards.

Yelp

www.yelp.com

Scope and Demographics

Yelp (Figure 5.11) helps consumers find all kinds of local businesses. Doctors and other healthcare providers are a small but growing component of the site. Founded in San Francisco in 2004, the site has a strong presence in major metropolitan areas across the United States, Canada, Europe, and Australia. Site statistics available in September 2012 showed that Yelp had a monthly average of nearly 80 million unique visitors in the second quarter of 2012. Since its inception, 30 million reviews have been contributed to the site. In addition, Yelp's mobile application was used on 7.2 million unique mobile devices on a monthly average basis during the same time period; approximately 40% of all Yelp searches are now done via mobile apps.

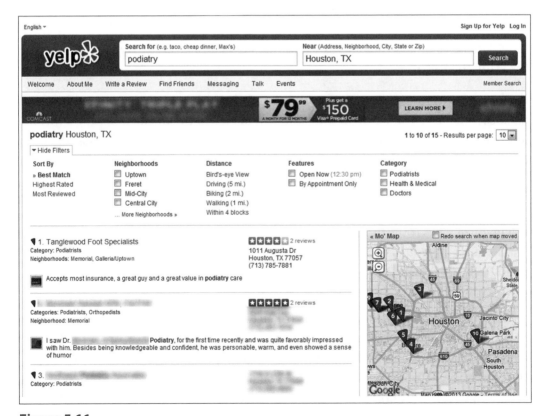

Figure 5.11

In the United States, 83% of Yelp users are under the age of 55, 65% have at least a college degree, and 86% earn in excess of $50,000 per year. Yelp does not break out its statistics for healthcare professionals.

How It Works

From the homepage, users seeking information on doctors can enter the specialty they are seeking or a provider's name and the area (by zip code) where they are seeking care. A search quickly produces a list of potential doctors, and more ways to filter the search results. A search for internal medicine doctors in San Diego, California, displayed a list of about 250 doctors. Because Yelp is a locally oriented site, it allows users to filter in a geographically granular way. Consumers can limit results to specific neighborhoods as well as biking, walking, or driving distance from a specific location. While the site allows for sorting results for the highest rated or most reviewed, it does not offer filtering by other attributes such as board certification or provider's sex, as most other doctor review sites do.

Clicking on the name of a doctor brings up a brief profile page. But because Yelp is oriented toward business details, it does not include detailed information on educational background or subspecialties. The profile contains the address, phone number, and any photos that have been posted either by the doctor or by a user of the site. The site includes an "Edit" button that allows anyone to make changes; but if the changes are not made by the site owner, Yelp will verify the changes before updating the listing.

If a user is searching for a specific doctor and that person is not included in Yelp's database, the user will be invited to add him or her to the business listings, but the user must have an account on Yelp to do so. Yelp also licenses information from third-party data providers that aggregate data from public records and other sources.

Beneath the basic business listing are the reviews that have been posted by users. Yelp's default sort order takes a number of factors into account. For example, the site will favor reviews from the user's friends and from other users they follow.

How Providers Are Rated

To write a review, users first select the number of stars (from one to five) to rate the doctor. Aside from general guidelines (one star = "eek methinks not" to five stars = "woohoo as good as it gets"), there are no specific rating categories on Yelp. Beneath the star rating is an open box for the reviewer to write a narrative review of up to 5001 characters. The site publishes some general guidelines for reviews, encouraging people to write only about firsthand experiences and to stay away from intellectual property violations, privacy breaches, conflicts of interest, and promotional content.

Yelp stresses that users should make reviews factually accurate and that reviews should reflect the most recent interaction the consumers have had with the business. So if a review is written by a patient with an ongoing relationship with your practice, Yelp would encourage that patient to update his or her review periodically to add new insights.

User trust and transparency are important to Yelp, so the site encourages users to provide details about themselves on their account profiles and to engage in honest conversations on the site. Yelp does not allow for fully anonymous reviews. Users who create an account on Yelp are given the opportunity to choose a nickname, but they cannot create or use an account for anyone other than themselves, provide an e-mail address other than their own, or create multiple accounts. Thus for any disputes that arise, Yelp knows the true identity of the reviewer.

Yelp has a controversial policy whereby some reviews are not posted. Those that don't make the cut are still available in a separate "Filtered Review" page. These sequestered reviews do not affect a doctor's overall star rating, but users can still read them by clicking on the link at the bottom of the doctor's profile page. The purpose of the filter is to establish an objective standard. Yelp admits that legitimate reviews are axed from time to time and that it may also miss some fake ones, too.

How Providers Can Interact with Yelp

Yelp encourages business owners to unlock their business account, which is a free and easy ("two minute") process. Physicians whose businesses appear on Yelp can communicate with patients both privately and publicly; track the user views on their business page; and add photos, a detailed practice description, up-to-date information, history, and specialties. Yelp also offers opportunities for businesses to offer "deals" (for which Yelp takes a cut). However, this service is unlikely to benefit healthcare professionals.

If you get a negative review, Yelp encourages you to contact the reviewer or post a public response in order to clear up any misunderstandings. It also urges you to bring the review to Yelp's attention if it violates the site's content guidelines (e.g., the reviewer admittedly describes a second-hand experience or uses a threat). Otherwise, Yelp will not remove or reorder bad reviews. Yelp believes it has checks and balances in its system that protect the integrity of the site for both consumers and business owners.

The site contains detailed guidelines on responding to both positive and negative reviews and responding publicly versus privately, but remember that you should be guided more by HIPAA policies and by the guidelines described in our chapter on professionalism (Chapter 7). Yelp's guidelines apply to all types of business and are not specific to the concerns of the healthcare community.

ZocDoc

www.zocdoc.com

Scope and Demographics

ZocDoc (Figure 5.12) started in 2007, and physician ratings have been an integral part of its services since the beginning. More than a ratings site, it offers a unique service

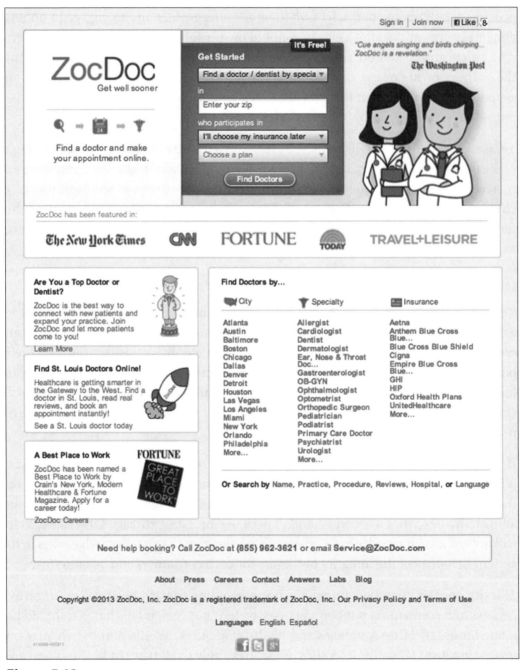

Figure 5.12

where patients can book appointments online 24/7. Think OpenTable for doctors' appointments. The company also offers an app for iPhone, Android, and Blackberry. ZocDoc allows patients to find a doctor who accepts their insurance and view that doctor's real-time availability.

As of September 2012, more than 1.7 million patients used ZocDoc each month. The service offers appointments with more than 148 different physician and dental specialties and is currently in 19 major metropolitan areas in the United States, with plans to expand nationwide in 2013. This represents a significant expansion in the past three years; in August 2010, ZocDoc was available in only four cities. On ZocDoc, 40% of appointments take place within 24 hours, 60% within three days; and 36% of ZocDoc appointments are booked while the doctor's office is closed. Preventive care is the type of procedure most booked through ZocDoc. The number of users per month increased nearly 850% between August 2010 and August 2012, and appointments booked through mobile apps grew 400% between July 2011 and July 2012.

How It Works

The ZocDoc homepage allows patients to search by location (city or zip code), specialty, and type of insurance accepted. The search results include a thumbnail photo, address, star rating, map, and appointment times available for each doctor listed. Ratings are tied to actual appointments, providing a measure of comfort for patients looking for real reviews and for doctors looking for reputable review sites. Patients must create an account before they make an appointment. Afterwards, they can return to the site to post a review. ZocDoc takes the patient back to an appointment summary page containing date and details of the appointment along with a thumbnail photo of the doctor. Clicking on the "Leave Feedback" button brings up a review form.

How Providers Are Rated

Patients are asked to rate the doctor by responding to several specific questions; they also have the option of submitting narrative comments. Ratings are done on a five-star scale, with one star meaning "never" and five stars meaning "highly recommended."

Patients are asked:

• Would you recommend this professional?
• How would you rate this professional's bedside manner?
• How long was the wait time in the office before you were seen? (For this question one star means "more than two hours" and five stars means "right away.")

Patients are also given the option to use their name and show their appointment in the review. Staff members at ZocDoc moderate all reviews before they are posted. For example, ZocDoc does not allow patients to put specific prices in their reviews. It believes that this aspect of the encounter reflects more on insurance companies than on the providers. It also will not publish profanity or offensive comments in the reviews. Only reviews written by actual, verified patients are allowed; ZocDoc checks to ensure that posted reviews are authentic.

How Providers Can Interact with ZocDoc

You pay a monthly fee to be included in ZocDoc. The company sells its service by promoting its ability to bring new patients to your office and to fill cancelled appointments. By being available 24/7 to patients looking for doctors' appointments and by linking to your practice management software, the service is able to provide real-time access to patients booking appointments.

ZocDoc consults with you to ensure that you are targeting the types of patients you want for your specialty. The company provides a widget that you can use on your practice website to drive traffic to the online booking site. A physician dashboard allows you to update your profile. A ZocDoc account manager works closely with you and your staff to create a profile and to ensure that you are well-represented and that the information is consistent.

Your profile includes a professional statement (written by you), a map of the practice site, the average star rating, and a photo. In addition, the listing provides your educational background, hospital affiliation, languages spoken, board certifications, awards and publications, and insurance accepted.

You are not able to comment on any posted review. Because all reviews are verified by a ZocDoc staff member before posting, disputed reviews are rare. However, if you contact the site about a review you believe to be inaccurate or fraudulent, ZocDoc will review it. First, ZocDoc will verify that the patient was actually seen by you. It will then discuss the issue with you. If there is factual accuracy in your claim, ZocDoc will remove the text of the review, but will retain the star rating that patient has given. ZocDoc believes that this process allows for "the patient's voice" to be heard.

There are three situations where ZocDoc will remove a review:

- It will not publish claims about the accuracy of your treatment and diagnosis, because ZocDoc believes these are factual matters that cannot be readily verified.
- Patients can state their opinion of whether your service came at a good price, but the site will not publish pricing specifics as mentioned earlier.
- ZocDoc will not post anything profane, vulgar, or otherwise offensive.

REFERENCES

1. Sepkowitz K. Doctor, Doctor, Give Me Reviews. Slate. November 28, 2008; www.slate.com/articles/health_and_science/medical_examiner/2008/11/doctor_doctor_give_me_reviews.html. Accessed November 8, 2012.

2. Strech D. Ethical principles for physician rating sites. *J Med Internet Res.* 2011;13:e113.

3. Fox S, Duggan M. Health Online. Pew Internet & American Life Project. 2013; http://pewinternet.org/Reports/2013/Health-online.aspx.

4. Insider Pages. Wikipedia, the free encyclopedia. http://en.wikipedia.org/wiki/Insider_Pages. Accessed December 17, 2012.

5. Blankenhorn D. Insiderpages launches doctor reviews. ZDNet. May 5, 2010; www.zdnet.com/blog/healthcare/insiderpages-launches-doctor-reviews/3608. Accessed December 17, 2012.

6. Collier R. Professionalism: logging on to tell your doctor off. *CMAJ.* 2012;184:E 629-630.

7. Gao GG, McCullough JS, Agarwal R, Jha AK. A changing landscape of physician quality reporting: analysis of patients' online ratings of their physicians over a 5-year period. *J Med Internet Res.* 2012;14:e38.

"Institutions are becoming naked, and if you're going to be naked . . . fitness is no longer optional. If you're going to be naked, you better get buff."

—DON TAPSCOTT

CHAPTER 6

Safeguarding Your Online Reputation

So, what's next? Now that you've taken the time to establish a digital footprint, it's time to develop a strategy for monitoring and maintaining your good reputation. If you are active in social media, you need to make sure your voice is heard. Moreover, responding to reviews (both good and bad), embracing constructive criticism, and encouraging patients to give good feedback are all key elements of protecting your online reputation.

MAKING SOCIAL MEDIA WORK FOR YOU: SEARCH ENGINE OPTIMIZATION

Discoverability is the new marketing. Previously, we encouraged you to bring social media full circle by publicizing your online presence in your practice. Web 2.0-compliant websites that facilitate sharing will significantly boost your search engine optimization (SEO) and keep the positive links on the first few pages of any search results.

If you have a practice website, you have probably heard about SEO. Broadly speaking, SEO refers to the way you market yourself or your practice on the Internet so that you show up high in search results for either your name, the name of your practice, or keywords describing your expertise (e.g., internal medicine doctor in Boston). Most keywords will be picked up from content on your website. In fact, much of SEO strategy centers on content marketing and maximizing the effectiveness of your website. Indeed, entire books have been written just on SEO. In the business world, it can make the difference between success and failure.

As it relates to reputation management, social media optimization (SMO) is perhaps an even more important element of your overall marketing and reputation management strategy. It means improving your online presence by focusing on social media communities. SMO is the process of improving the discoverability and usability of your presence in social media. Since most online experiences begin with a search engine, this is clearly an important component of your online reputation and can be dealt with separately from website optimization. So, for instance, if you are part of a group practice, you can focus on SMO to build your own brand within the practice and within the community at large.

As this book is being written (fall 2012), a huge increase in social sharing on the Web is changing the way many search results are reported. For example, Google now integrates numerous social sites into its search results. Information and links that have been shared by the searcher's social network through sites such as Facebook and Twitter will now rank high. This development could be an enormous change for the search process in the future. The trend here is that people who share information online, and build large social networks, are more likely to see themselves ranked high in search engine results.

Google also made some significant changes to its search algorithms in 2012 that will benefit doctors who choose to blog. Its Panda and Penguin algorithmic updates penalize low-quality sites and SEO techniques that violate Google's Webmaster Guidelines. The result is that sites rich in content are rewarded. Websites that have been stuffed with numerous keywords in the hopes of raising visibility on a results page will be at a disadvantage here while high-quality sites that regularly update their content (e.g., through a blog) will have much to gain. Linking to other reputable sources of information (e.g., institutions, associations, colleagues) will also make your blog more credible in the eyes of Google.

You can use many of the principles of SMO by following the guidelines under the "Maximizing" heading for each of the six major social media channels described in Chapter 4. To further help you make the most of these outlets and build your online reputation, below are some tips to keep in mind as you work with each site:

- Make sure your presence is consistent across social media platforms—use the same name, photograph, and logo to build brand identity.
- Titles and tags are key.
- Content is king. The more useful your content is and the more it is targeted to the interests of your patient population, the more likely it is to rank high in search engines. If your content isn't of sufficient quality to attract good natural links, it doesn't matter how "optimized" that content is.
- Incorporate images and/or videos into your social media communications.
- Post or update often. Activity levels, especially recent activity, drive search engine results.
- If you have a website, use Google Analytics, a free tool, to track website activity. What keywords are visitors entering in a search box that leads them to you? What questions are they asking? Make sure the titles and tags in any new content you create match those words or answer the questions that patients may use in a search.

- Make it easy for people to share information about you and your practice by including links to all your social media sites on each of your sites. For example, make sure your LinkedIn page has links to your Facebook page and Twitter account.
- You do not need to buy ads on Google to be visible on the first page of search results. Most users prioritize the importance of organic search results over ads.

PATIENT SATISFACTION IS NOW A VITAL METRIC

Hospitals and practices have conducted patient satisfaction surveys for years. Press Ganey is one well-known company that works with hospitals and physician groups, performing formal surveys and producing case studies, webinars, and other resources designed to help medical practices improve patient satisfaction.

Over the past several years, patient satisfaction has gained increasing attention from executives across the healthcare industry and from the federal government. Hospitals began reporting their Hospital Consumer Assessment of Healthcare Providers and Systems (HCAHPS) scores in 2008; and starting October 1, 2012, Medicare has based its reimbursements in part on these measures. These new rules have raised the stakes for patient satisfaction surveys. As a measure of quality, patient satisfaction is highly complex and controversial. Although it has been linked to positive outcomes in some studies, others have shown the opposite result. Debate on this issue will go on for a long time, and the relationship between patient satisfaction and reimbursement will evolve as more data become available.

A full discussion of the ramifications of patient satisfaction is outside the scope of this book. What's important here is its increased visibility and, thus, its greater relevance to your reputation. Because of the emphasis being placed on patient satisfaction today, it can no longer simply be relegated to periodic surveys or ignored altogether. The growth of the ratings business online has made it easier for patients to describe their healthcare experiences in detail and to express their satisfaction—or lack thereof. Increasingly, the online rating sites are the places where patients' opinions will be aired.

Here's another reason to embrace patient satisfaction ratings—the metrics used are similar to those already used by the Centers for Medicare & Medicaid Services (CMS) and are sure to affect individual physicians in the future. They are the shape of things to come. Why not address these issues now?

Soliciting patient feedback, listening to patients talk about both their positive and negative experiences, and using those observations to improve your practice is a good way to safeguard your reputation. A study of more than 5000 primary care patients a few years ago identified seven traits of physician excellence that directly affected patient satisfaction as reflected in their ratings of physicians: access, communication, personality and demeanor of provider, quality of medical care processes, care continuity, quality of healthcare facilities, and office staff.[1]

A more recent report focused on empathy as another driver of positive physician ratings. A group at Massachusetts General Hospital studied the effectiveness of brief empathy training modules for resident physicians. The researchers found "statistically significant improvement in patient perception and ratings of physician empathy."[2] Another study showed empathy to be positively correlated with patient outcomes. In a 2011 study of patients with diabetes, researchers found that patients who had rated their doctors highly on empathy scores were most likely to have good control of both hemoglobin A1c and low-density lipoprotein cholesterol levels.[3]

A 2012 study of baby boomers (those born between 1946 and 1964) contains an interesting finding from this increasingly large segment of the patient population. Of the 400 people surveyed, 86% said their patient experience would be better if the doctor talked to them about changing their behavior rather than immediately prescribing a drug.[4] (See Patient Satisfaction Tips on page 157 for more recommendations gleaned from various organizations and studies.)

Other industries have seen a direct correlation between revenue and positive customer experience. Forrester Research estimates that above-average customer satisfaction scores can save health insurance plans significant revenue.[5] The same metrics are becoming more important to the bottom line of individual medical practices as well and will become more so as the government puts its trust in scores as a reliable indicator of quality care.

In some respects, the future is already here. Recall that in Chapter 1, we noted that general societal trends ultimately affect healthcare as well—it just takes a little longer. The era of empowered consumers, where online interactivity has allowed them to take greater control over their lives, is an excellent example of this phenomenon. A recent survey of 6000 adults found that patient satisfaction is more important than price, especially in healthcare. In a report released in July 2012, PricewaterhouseCoopers (PwC) Health Research Institute compared consumer attitudes in banking, hospitality, airline, and retail industries with their experiences and opinions in healthcare.[6]

PwC found some similarities in consumer expectations of healthcare as compared with other industries—convenience and speed. But the differences are more telling. The survey showed that price is not a top inducement for choosing a healthcare provider. Only 8% of respondents ranked price as the primary driver of their decision, compared with 69% for leisure airline travel, 55% for retail, and even 50% for selecting a health insurer. Instead, 42% of consumers surveyed ranked personal *experience* as the number one criterion in choosing a healthcare provider. Individual consumers also rely on their personal networks and peer recommendations. Overall, the study found that 72% of

PATIENT SATISFACTION TIPS

1. Understand your patients' preferences. Do they want phone calls, e-mails, or texts for appointment reminders? Adjust your communications practices accordingly.
2. Focus solutions on transparency, knowledge, and convenience. Consider offering mobile check-in, digital appointment reminders, medical reminders, price comparison tools, and free Wi-Fi.
3. Take advantage of multiple access points to educate and engage consumers. Provide in-person customer support for those who prefer it and virtual support for people who prefer that approach.
4. Train staff to welcome each patient with a smile, declutter the front desk, refrain from having food and beverages in sight, keep personal conversations quiet and to a minimum, and dress appropriately for the office.
5. Grant employees authority to change the customer experience. Train all staff on how to talk to patients, review staff performance, and share stories to improve the patient experience.
6. Don't keep patients waiting more than 15 minutes. If you are running behind schedule, consider sending patients a text message to alert them.
7. Talk to patients about behavioral changes they can make to improve their health.
8. Be proactive—go beyond the transaction. Train staff to acknowledge difficult situations and apologize.
9. Give patients a printed summary of their visit, including diagnosis and action plans.
10. Communication is key—make eye contact, involve patients in discussions of treatment options, and express complex information in layman's terms.
11. Keep the office environment attractive—have current and diverse magazines, clean furniture, healthy plants, straightened pictures and posters, music or TV that is not too loud, and clean restrooms.
12. Seek customer feedback.

Sources: Catalyst Healthcare Research[4]; PwC Health Research Institute[6]; Stewart EE, McMillen M.[19]

consumers ranked the reputation of the healthcare provider and personal experience as the top driver for choosing a provider.[6] Other important findings include:

• **The attitude of the healthcare team matters.** PwC found that, when compared with the banking and hospitality industries, staff attitude was twice as important in healthcare provider decisions.

• **Apologies are viewed positively.** Healthcare consumers said they would be willing to go back to a provider who apologizes.

• **"Ideal" experiences drive change.** More than a third of consumers said they would change providers or insurance plans if they offered an "ideal experience," defined in the study as nonclinical aspects of care, such as "convenience, amenities, and customer service."[6]

See what several doctors have to say about the concept of patient satisfaction today. Steve Bates, MD, a plastic surgeon and founder of DocsVox, writes[7]:

> In my mind, the whole concept of patient satisfaction is about having a conversation with our patients to determine what they think we are doing well and what they think we need to improve upon. It is about having that conversation in a meaningful and transparent way that makes our patients believe we are actually listening to them.
>
> It isn't about some number that needs to be benchmarked and then branded on us like a scarlet letter. So why aren't we having this conversation with the tools of communication that we use in every other aspect of our life and work? Why don't we integrate email, cloud computing, social media, mobile technology and modern data analytics into these surveys? And why don't we link them to our EMRs and our practice web pages and truly integrate them into our practices? These things are all possible with technology that is already almost a decade old!

Stephen Schimpff, MD, an internist, professor of medicine and public policy, former CEO of the University of Maryland Medical Center, and author of *The Future of Medicine—Megatrends in Healthcare* (Thomas Nelson, 2007) and *The Future of Health Care Delivery* (Potomac Books, 2012), writes[8]:

> Consumerism is becoming—finally—more and more of a driver of change. Patients are coming to want and *expect* to be treated like a valued customer. Like the movie where he shouted "I can't take it anymore," now "the patient is no longer willing to be patient anymore." What do the patients want? They want service, good service. They increasingly understand that quality and safety are not ideal so they are looking for and expecting high levels of quality & safety. Perhaps the most important one of all is respect, respect for their person, confidentially, and the quality of their care. But also patients want convenience & responsiveness. They don't want to have to travel long distances, wait long times in the "waiting room," nor be put on indefinite telephone hold. They want interaction by email and other electronic methods. And finally, patients increasingly expect to close the information gap—they expect the playing field between patient and doctor to be much more level in the future.

SET UP ALERTS

Because search engines give priority to recently posted information, it pays to keep an eye on your online presence at all times. In fact, I recommend that every healthcare

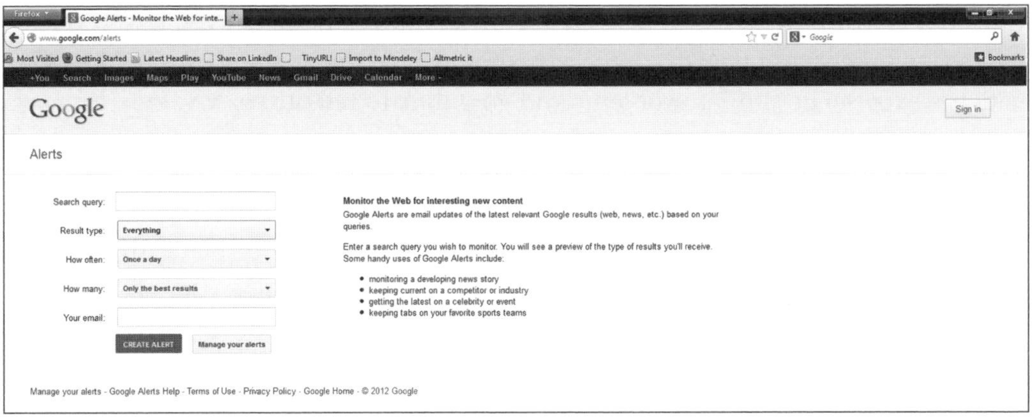

Figure 6.1

professional Google their name at least once a week to see what comes up. Remember, more of your patients are doing exactly that. One way to automate this process is to sign up for a Google Alert (www.google.com/alerts) as shown in Figure 6.1.

In this form, enter your name or your practice's name into the search query field, along with an e-mail address. Use all forms of your name to ensure that you see all results. You will be automatically notified whenever Google sees a mention of you. It's a very simple process that allows you to know if new information has been posted about you without having to monitor numerous sites daily. The advantage to these alerts is that you can get immediate reports, take a quick glance to see if it's important or something you need to investigate further or respond to, and simply delete. You may be surprised at how often your name appears on Google.

You can also set up alerts on Facebook, LinkedIn, YouTube, and Twitter to notify you when messages are posted. Some of the review sites may have an alert option as well, but you first have to claim your profile listing on the site.

THE SCOPE OF ONLINE REVIEWS

As patient care transitions to team-based models, every member of the team is central to the physician's reputation. That includes doctors, nurses, physician assistants, medical assistants, and, just as important, receptionists. In fact, the most common complaints in online reviews center on nonclinical issues such as the attitude of the front desk staff, the décor in the office, or the lack of good parking. These aspects of the patient's experience aren't foremost in a doctor's mind when he or she considers the patient. But you can be sure they are an integral part of the patient's experience with your practice.

Consider all reviews carefully. Do you see any common themes? Even if only one or two reviews mention a negative issue, you should heed the warning now before other patients experience similar problems and go online to tell others.

Many physicians don't look at online reviews unless they learn about a negative review or have had a review adversely affect their practice. The current review structure is far from perfect. Many of us have heard horror stories about blatantly negative reviews that almost certainly were not posted by actual patients. After all, what's to stop the disgruntled ex-employee, the vindictive ex-spouse, or even the misguided doctor down the street from posting comments that could harm your reputation? In short, nothing. Free speech is a guaranteed right in the United States. Defamation is exceedingly difficult to prove in today's online world, where *opinions* rule.

FOCUS ON THE POSITIVE

As unsettling as this environment may seem, let's focus on the majority of reviews, not the outliers. As we stated in the first chapter, several studies concluded that, in fact, most online reviews of physicians are positive. Let's look at more evidence.

The rating site DrScore conducted an analysis of 15,000 ratings posted from 2004 to 2010 and reported its findings in the journal *Health Outcomes Research in Medicine*. The study showed that the average physician rating was 9.3 on a 10-point scale. Even more noteworthy: 70% of physicians had perfect scores![9] You probably won't hear about these types of reviews in the popular press. The media thrive on negative news. But the evidence should convince you that not only are the risks of negative reviews overstated, but you actually have much to gain from embracing online reviews.

We hope the previous chapter on the major review sites has encouraged you to at least go to those sites to ensure that basic information about you and your practice is correct. It's a sad fact that much of the data on those sites are outdated. If your information is current and complete, you're a step ahead of many of your colleagues.

INVITE YOUR PATIENTS TO WRITE REVIEWS

Patient recommendations can carry more weight with other patients than any traditional marketing campaigns you may have. Use them to your advantage. Link the reviews from a ratings site back to your website. Even if you already have testimonials on your site, outside reviews can increase credibility.

The best way to get positive reviews is to ask patients to post reviews about their experiences in your office. One way to do this is to give them a card at checkout that steers them to a specific review site, or you might direct them to choose from among several review sites that you have preselected and trust. Your front office staff can encourage patients to give feedback. A sign posted in a prominent place within the office can reinforce your message that you want your patients to be heard and that you value their input.

It's good practice to enter a quick response, even if it's just to say "thank you," to patients who have praised you. To comply with HIPAA, ask patients for their permission to publicly respond to their review online. When you respond to patient reviews, you are letting them know that their opinion matters to you. Over time, and coupled with other steps to get more reviews, you will build a solid reputation that won't be diminished by one or two negative reviews.

Read how New Orleans-based urologist Neil Baum, MD, hands out cards (Figure 6.2) to patients encouraging them to write online reviews, so he can use the reviews to shape his online reputation:

What are physicians' most precious possessions? Some might answer that it is their patients. Others might respond it is the training and education that physicians have obtained to practice their craft. But the real answer is that it's the physicians' reputation. Doctors live and die by their reputations. These reputations take years to build but are so fragile that they can crumble in a matter of seconds.

A colleague called me after he saw an unflattering review about me on an online website. The reviewer, who was anonymous, referred to me as technologically advanced but more motivated to increase my income by performing too many diagnostic tests.

It is my observation that most online reviews of physicians are positive, and most physicians have five or fewer reviews on any one site. Let's face it, even the most charming, charismatic, and experienced physician cannot possibly satisfy every patient who walks through the door.

The most successful practices acquire reviews organically, a technique that is often achieved through quality customer service and outstanding patient care. To encourage a steady flow, you can administer a process to encourage your most satisfied, loyal patients to review your practice. Make the process simple. Hand patients a review card (see mine, Figure 6.2) as they leave your office with easy steps for leaving a review online. A patient pleased with your service will be happy to take five minutes to review your practice. Acquire 5 to 10 reviews monthly, and within a year's time you will have generated enough positive reviews to negate any damaging comments that will inevitably emerge from time to time.

Now, I have a robust Internet presence with my name and my practice appearing at the top of the search engine response page when "urologist" plus "New Orleans" is typed into Google. By far most of the reviews of my practice are positive, and I have balanced the rare negative response with numerous and plentiful positive responses.

Patients are seeking and leaving reviews about you and your practice online. Do not let one disgruntled patient ruin your reputation. My advice is to take an active role and generate positive reviews to drown out any negative remarks made by the occasional patient.

Neil Baum, MD

Urologist

New Orleans, Louisiana

www.neilbaum.com

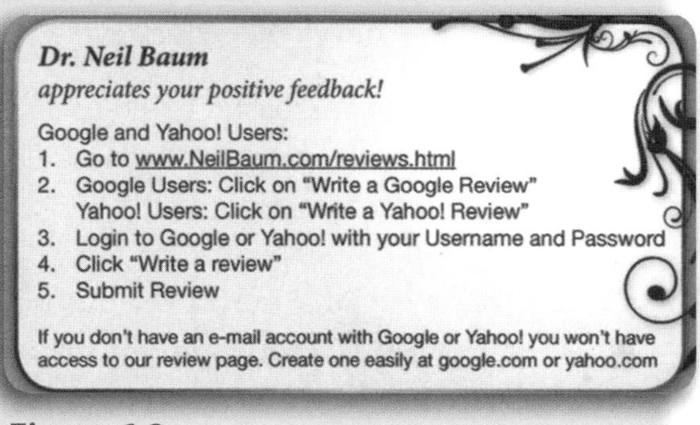

Dr. Neil Baum *appreciates your positive feedback!*

Google and Yahoo! Users:
1. Go to www.NeilBaum.com/reviews.html
2. Google Users: Click on "Write a Google Review"
   Yahoo! Users: Click on "Write a Yahoo! Review"
3. Login to Google or Yahoo! with your Username and Password
4. Click "Write a review"
5. Submit Review

If you don't have an e-mail account with Google or Yahoo! you won't have access to our review page. Create one easily at google.com or yahoo.com

Figure 6.2

You'll notice that Baum's card gently alludes to asking for positive reviews. Other practices are more neutral, simply asking patients to give their feedback, good or bad, to these online sites and letting the proverbial chips fall where they may. As noted previously, multiple studies have found that most patients rate their doctors favorably online. Your patients are probably no exception.

USE REVIEWS TO IMPROVE YOUR PRACTICE

What about reviews that are less than stellar? Use negative reviews to improve your practice. Read them carefully. These ratings provide a sense of transparency. They can tell you how patients feel about their experiences in your care. Often, when patients leave the exam room, you do not know what they thought about the nurse, the front office staff, or the parking situation, but all of these factors affect their experience. I have read many reviews, and I get the sense that some patients are frustrated with our healthcare system. They are frustrated that they have to wait weeks or months to see a doctor. They are frustrated that they never get a copy of their results when they have blood drawn or get an x-ray.

More recently, they are frustrated with doctors looking at computer screens or tablets, rather than looking at the patient who is talking to them. Consider this anecdote from New Jersey-based oncologist James Salwitz, MD, who recalls what a patient said to him about computers in the exam room[10]:

> When we go to see the doctor, he stares at the computer. He does not look at us. Most of the time, the doctor is not even listening to us. He just sits there typing at the keyboard, gaping at the screen. If he had been listening when my wife talked about the pain, then he would have stopped the drug . . . All you doctors have become nothing but computers.

Focus on the constructive criticism of a bad review. Analyze it to determine why the patient is unhappy. Are the issues mentioned ones you've heard before? Are there things you could do differently to improve situations like these?

I've made changes in my own practice on the basis of this type of feedback. I make sure I offer more same-day appointments. I ensure that patients receive a copy of their lab test results. I no longer bring a laptop computer or tablet into the exam room because I am looking at patients in the eye when I'm talking to them. Online reviews have helped me change my practice, and I believe they have made me a better doctor.

One study looked at tens of thousands of these reviews and distilled two factors that impacted these ratings the most[11]:

- Wait times longer than 15 minutes; and
- Visit length shorter than 10 minutes.

To maximize your online ratings, keep these numbers in mind.

In 2011, Press Ganey published a report that found the average satisfaction score for wait times up to 15 minutes was 94.3 on a 100-point scale. If the wait exceeded 15 minutes, the score fell by nearly four points; and for waits more than an hour, scores fell to 86.1.[11]

Family physician Michael Woo-Ming, MD, explains how medicine is now a customer service business:

> **Let's face it. Most physicians and healthcare professionals are too busy. Yet as a doctor myself, I know firsthand how you want to do as much as you can for your patients, such as making sure prescriptions are called in or working in an urgent appointment.**
>
> **Then why do most doctors ignore what's being said about them on the Internet?**
>
> **Recently, I was chatting with a physician who had received an unflattering review on a public forum. She knew it was there (most providers do), yet chose the defensive tactic, "Oh people don't believe anything on the Internet." Unfortunately, it is easy to make sweeping generalizations; but**

ignoring the complaint sends a message to most prospective and current patients that if a gripe is posted online, then the review must be true! According to a recent consumer study, one of three customers who have a negative experience take the time to post their opinion online. The fact is, you can be one of the most outstanding physicians in the world, but most patients won't take the time to post something positive.

And that is the issue in a nutshell. In medicine, we may have different specialties, but we are all in the customer service business.

Take the time to understand what is being written about you online and why. Can you identify who wrote the post? Don't forget your ancillary staff is a part of who you are as a doctor and will have more impact than you might think. Are you and your staff being abrupt to patients? Are patient waiting times too long? Could a problem have been handled with better communication? In our experience, most negative reviews start as a misunderstanding.

Periodically follow up with your patients through e-mail. Proactively encourage patients to fill out testimonials and online forums. Improving online physician reputation management starts in the office.

Michael Woo-Ming, MD, MPH
Chief Executive Officer
RepMD
Escondido, California
http://repmd.com

HOW TO RESPOND TO NEGATIVE REVIEWS

Even though most online reviews are likely to be positive, remember that they also reflect the patient's overall experience in your care. As discussed in previous chapters, these reviews often focus on nonclinical issues not directly related to the doctor. But those comments are no less important to your reputation.

Yet, you're a physician. Your profession has different standards from other types of businesses that are reviewed online. Some rules for reputation management don't apply to you. For instance, Yelp encourages businesses to "create a Yelp Deal" by offering discounts to customers who find the business on their site, to "turn Yelp visitors into paying customers." They also advise business owners to message customers, and "join the conversation regarding a business." Obviously, these guidelines cannot be used by medical practitioners to manage their online reputations on Yelp or any other review site.

Online reputation companies often try to bury bad reviews by creating more positive information to improve the search rankings of a business. Some of their strategies include publishing numerous press releases with positive news about the business or individual, and creating multiple websites about various products and services of a business as a way to divert attention away from the negative reviews and give the business more positive visibility in search results. Most medical practices do not lend themselves to these types of solutions.

Doctors actually have numerous options for responding to patient reviews, according to Eric Goldman, professor of law at Santa Clara University School of Law. He has written extensively on legal issues relating to online rating sites:

- **Respond generally.** Most negative reviews relate to nonclinical aspects of the practice such as parking, wait times, out-of-date magazines, or staff attitude.[12] Doctors can respond to those issues directly in the review site without violating privacy laws. Explain these aspects of your practice without confirming or denying that the reviewer was your patient. Explain how you run your practice in general terms, but refrain from publically talking about the specifics of any one patient's experience.
- **Address individuals offline.** Responding to negative reviews that criticize bedside manner or question medical judgment should never be done in a public forum. Some sites, like Yelp, allow providers to privately respond to patient reviews. You may take the opportunity to do so. But it's better to take this conversation offline. A standard response to call the office to further discuss the concern is appropriate.
- **Ask for permission to reply.** Finally, you can ask patients for their permission to publically reply to their reviews or post an apology. Once you have their written consent, a public response or apology can show others in the forum that you are listening to patients and taking steps to address their concerns. Doing this potentially turns the negative situation of a bad review into a more constructive experience.[13]

In a *New England Journal of Medicine* perspective piece published in October 2012, "Why Doctors Prescribe Opioids to Known Opioid Abusers," Stanford psychiatrist Anna Lembke, MD, explains the various pressures doctors face when patients ask them to prescribe controlled substances. One is patient ratings:

> The prioritization of the subjective experience of pain has been reinforced by the modern practice of regularly assessing patient satisfaction. Patients fill out surveys about the care they receive, which commonly include questions about how adequately their providers have addressed their pain. Doctors' clinical skills may also be evaluated on for-profit doctor-grading websites for the world to see.

> Doctors who refuse to prescribe opioids to certain patients out of concern about abuse are likely to get a poor rating from those patients . . .

> . . . When I asked a physician colleague who regularly treats pain how he deals with the problem of using opioids in patients who he knows are abusing them, he said, "Sometimes I just have to do the right thing and refuse to prescribe them, even if I know they're going to go on Yelp and give me a bad rating." [14]

Online ratings should never get in the way of practicing good medicine. If a physician gets a bad review because he was "doing the right thing" by refusing an inappropriate request for a controlled substance, use the principles described above.

Take the conversation offline by using a standard response to call the office. Do so without confirming or denying that the reviewer is your patient. If the patient is known to you, you may ask for his or her written permission to respond publicly, where you can then address the patient's concerns and perhaps explain your motive to stem the epidemic of prescription drug abuse.

Obviously, posting responses is reactive and shouldn't be your only strategy for combating negative reviews. Those reviews will live a long time online, and could become fodder for malpractice attorneys or could impact your ability to sell your practice. In other words, they can haunt you for a long time.

Be proactive instead. Consider the patient's experience and make sure that the customer service aspects of your practice meet acceptable standards as part of the new definition of professionalism in medicine. Once you excel in service, encourage more patients to review you online. In the end, any negative reviews will appear to be outliers.

DON'T STUFF THE BALLOT BOX

The *Journal of General Internal Medicine* study that analyzed online reviews also found that some doctors even wrote reviews about themselves. One was quoted as saying, "Every anonymous review I've written on myself has been glowing." The study also showed that doctors may not be very good at writing reviews pretending to be from a patient's perspective because they often used terminology not widely known to the lay public.[12]

Recall the article from Slate, mentioned in Chapter 4, where physician Kent Sepkowitz, MD, writes about the flaws in online rating systems. He also writes about how he boosted his own reviews after seeing his ratings:

> I was reviewed on one of the freebie sites, DrScore.com—and, um, someone out there doesn't like me. All of my measures fell short—my exam, timeliness,

treatment, even my staff. So I did what any normal American male under e-assault would do. I stuffed the ballot box. I pretended to be a patient of mine and lied about my age, gender, how often I see me, and the reason I was seeing me. I talked up my friendly attitude and thoroughness, gushed over the oodles of time I spent examining me, and declared my overall treatment a success. Not to limit the kudos, I also gave high marks to parking availability by my office . . . With my unceasing selfishness campaign, I was able to hike my scores to levels that would make my mother and even my mother-in-law proud.[15]

But stuffing the ballot box really isn't a good idea because the rating site administrators aren't stupid. If they find too many positive reviews coming from one computer, they may simply delete those reviews altogether. So rather than write glowing reviews about yourself, let the patients do it—the reviews probably will be better than you think.

LAWSUITS ARE NOT THE ANSWER

It's not easy to remove a bad online rating. Yelp spokesperson Chantelle Karl says, "If we are contacted by a doctor or dentist with a take-down notice based on a contract restricting the patient's right to free speech, we will not honor the request (and will inform them of that)."[16] Most of the other rating sites profiled in this book have procedures in place that could result in their removing a negative review if it is found to be fraudulent or otherwise violates a site's terms of service. But the burden of proof rests largely with the doctor. Fighting a negative review can take months of gathering information and negotiating with the ratings site before any action is taken. Unless the site finds a specific policy violation or fraud, it is unlikely to remove a negative review because doing so would infringe on a patient's right to free speech.

Some healthcare providers have gone to court over negative ratings that they believe are unfair. This practice is generally not recommended because a lawsuit is not likely to produce a successful outcome. In addition, it is extremely time consuming and expensive. I am not aware of very many lawsuits where a physician or other healthcare provider has successfully sued an online rating site to remove a negative review.

Some physicians have sued the patients themselves. One of the most well-known cases involved Minnesota neurologist David McKee, MD. In 2009, he was caring for a stroke patient. The patient's son wasn't very happy with the care being given to his father, and he made his feelings known in a public way—he posted negative comments about McKee on online rating sites and notified the state medical board as well. Obviously, McKee wasn't pleased to read the son's comments. He decided to fight back. He claimed that the patient's son defamed him and interfered with his business by making false statements to the American Academy of Neurology, to the American Neurological Association, and on physician rating sites, among others. He sued the son for defamation. Initially, the court ruled against McKee and dismissed the lawsuit.

The physician filed an appeal. The Appeals Court overruled the lower court's decision. After four years, countless hours, and large expenditures, the case was dismissed by the Minnesota Supreme Court in January 2013.[17]

Perhaps McKee realized he had nothing more to lose when it came to his online reputation, but this certainly makes the situation immeasurably worse. What's worse is the media firestorm surrounding this case. This phenomenon is known as the Streisand Effect, where an attempt to censor or remove information online backfires, and the opposite effect actually occurs. Instead of being deleted, the situation gets widespread publicity, and is often shared across the Internet in a very short timeframe. (The name "Streisand Effect" is derived from a lawsuit filed by Barbra Streisand over the online posting of an aerial photo of her house.) Whenever McKee's name is put into a search engine, the publicity generated by his lawsuit will be featured prominently in the search results. By suing the patient, not only is the outcome of the suit in doubt, but he actually made the situation much worse.

No matter what kind of merit you think a case might have, doctors who sue patients for online ratings are going to lose in the more influential court of public opinion. Better that doctors take some slanderous lumps online, and instead, encourage more of their patients to rate them. The ensuing positive ratings that most will receive will drown out whatever vitriol is present.

GAG ORDERS DON'T WORK EITHER

Attempts to prevent negative reviews by using "gag order" contracts with patients have also not proved to be an effective solution to manage online patient reviews. A company called Medical Justice began offering contracts of this type to physicians. Originally founded in 2001 to help protect doctors from malpractice suits, in 2007 it started offering its members a contract to give to patients called "Mutual Agreement to Maintain Privacy." These types of agreements are widely referred to as gag orders. The patient is required to agree upfront that he or she will not publish derogatory commentary or reviews, *even anonymously*. The forms further require the patient to transfer the copyright on any future reviews he or she might write about that medical professional. Theoretically, if the doctor or dentist doesn't like the review, he or she can take it down, claiming copyright infringement.

But consider what happened to a patient who signed this contract. Robert Lee, a technology writer in New York City, awoke one morning with excruciating tooth pain. After finding a dentist through an online search, he was asked to sign the contract before the dentist would treat him. Because Lee was in severe pain and needed immediate treatment, he signed the agreement. During the next few months, Lee got into a billing dispute with the dentist over problems he had getting the necessary insurance paperwork from the dentist's office. As he became more frustrated with the lack of resolution to his dispute, he wrote about his experience on Yelp and on DoctorBase.

The dentist wrote to Lee, demanding that he take down the posts or face a lawsuit for breach of contract. After the review sites refused to take down the negative reviews, the dentist claimed that a copyright clause gave her ownership and started charging Lee fines of $100 for each day the criticism remained online. Charges had reached over $4000 when Lee, with the help of advocacy group Public Citizen, filed a class action suit against the dentist.[18]

Shortly thereafter, Medical Justice advised its 3500 clients to stop using the contracts. The company has since taken a different approach to online reviews, offering services for doctors to monitor their online reputation, respond to ratings, and post verified patient reviews online.

Often, privacy agreements are created under the guise of giving patients additional protection above what is mandated by HIPAA. But most experts believe it is unethical for doctors to ask patients to sign away their rights before medical care is given. In addition, legal experts say that the copyright claims are not enforceable and would not stand up in court. RateMDs, one of the more popular online rating sites, has a feature called "Wall of Shame" on its site. Patients are invited to add to this list names of doctors who use gag contracts, which is visible to anyone using the site.

In the final analysis, it's just not worth it for physicians to take these sorts of steps to protect themselves from negative online reviews. In fact, many people believe that your reputation is more credible if you have mixed reviews. As long as most reviews are positive, potential patients will see the negatives for what they are—one person's opinion.

OUTSOURCING REPUTATION MANAGEMENT

Online consultants offer services in areas that everyone really should know themselves, but often healthcare professionals are too busy to manage their online reputation. If you want to outsource this aspect of practice management, reputation consultants can be a good alternative. They use many of the same strategies and techniques that are covered in this book. In addition, they may have specialized expertise in SEO or in creating biographical information and other content that could enable you to get a better online profile quickly.

Generally, reputation management companies have two approaches. The proactive approach is used to build content that is associated with your name so that when your name is Googled that content will rank high in search results. This content might be in the form of a website or blog. Companies and consultants also offer a reactive approach where, if you already have negative information associated with your name, they will help you build content to rank above the negative ratings in search engine results. However, this reactive approach is much more difficult to accomplish and can take much longer to implement. Ideally, you want to build content before anything else is written about you. Remember, you have 100% control over the content you create and zero control over content created by others about you.

A wide array of reputation management companies exists to offer services to all types of business owners trying to grow their business or combat negative reviews and to job seekers looking to impress potential employers. Not surprisingly in the current environment where everyone Googles everybody, the number of reputation management companies has grown exponentially. While these companies can provide valuable services to healthcare professionals, it pays to choose wisely and avoid scam artists that promise more than they can deliver, make unwarranted claims, and just want to make a quick buck.

How do you select a company? First, ask yourself what you need a reputation management company to do for you. Do you want to start or increase your social media presence? Do you want to find ways to get more positive reviews on rating sites? Do you want someone to monitor rating sites and other social media and give you periodic reports? Do you have negative reviews and want to minimize their effect on your practice? Once you've determined what you need from a reputation management company, start exploring options online. Keyword searches could include: "doctor reputation management"; "physician reputation management"; and "online reputation management doctors."

Here are some tips for assessing a potential partner:

- **Verify credibility.** Before contacting a company, check out *its* reputation. After all, you're considering putting your reputation in the company's hands. Check out the management team. Does the website have bios of the company leaders that show what the team has done in the past? If the site does not have the names and photos of its leaders, consider that a red flag that may indicate a lack of integrity or authenticity.
- **Get a referral.** Ask friends or colleagues who have worked with reputation companies about their experiences. These need not be just other physicians. Reputation companies work with professionals in other fields—business, law, etc.—and the techniques used are similar.

- **Ask your website consultant.** If you work with a website developer or marketing consultant, it's possible that he or she can provide some of the SEO services to enhance your online visibility. If not, he or she might be able to refer you to a trustworthy source. Some medical marketing consultants also now incorporate reputation management into their work.

- **Experience counts.** What experience does the company have in reputation management and with healthcare in particular? Start by looking at how long the company has been in business but don't be too concerned if it's only a few years—this is a new field! Many reputation management companies are outgrowths of marketing companies whose leaders have expertise in Web marketing and SEO, skills that are necessary to tackle online reputation management.

- **Check out the company's work.** Some companies proudly display case studies on their site. You should not hesitate to ask for a reference if you want to learn more about how a company has helped a doctor. Much of the work is done in strict confidence, and you may not find many details on the site. The company should also be willing to share some stats with you on the results it has achieved for others.

- **Get a proposal.** Before signing a contract, you should get a thorough proposal. The company should detail its strategic plan for managing your reputation along with the amount of time that implementing the plan is expected to take and the cost. You should also ask about guarantees. What does it guarantee and in what time frame? Is there any sort of money-back guarantee?

- **Know what you're paying for.** Prices vary widely for reputation management. Some companies will do an initial evaluation at no charge. This approach could allow you to become comfortable working with the staff before you actually spend any money. It also enables the company to make a more accurate assessment of the time it will take to establish or repair your reputation. Some companies will also offer a tiered-pricing structure so that you can select the level of services you need. ⊞

REFERENCES

1. Anderson R, Barbara A, Feldman S. What patients want: a content analysis of key qualities that influence patient satisfaction. *J Med Pract Manage*. 2007; 22:255-261.

2. Reiss H. Teaching Empathy Can Improve Patient Satisfaction. Vital Signs. Massachusetts Medical Society. October 2012; www.massmed.org/AM/Template.cfm?Section=Home6&CONTENTID=77303&TEMPLATE=/CM/ContentDisplay.cfm. Accessed November 14, 2012.

3. Hojat M, Louis DZ, Markham FW, et al. Physicians' empathy and clinical outcomes for diabetic patients. *Acad Med*. 2011;86:359-364.

4. Catalyst Healthcare Research. Innovative Ways to Improve the Patient Experience. Nashville; 2012; www.catalysthealthcareresearch.com/whatsreasonable-publicstudy/innovative-ways-to-improve-the-patient-experience. Accessed November 14, 2012.

5. Forrester Research. The Business Impact of Customer Experience. 2012.

6. PwC Health Research Institute. Customer Experience in Healthcare: The Moment of Truth. July 2012; www.pwc.com/es_MX/mx/publicaciones/archivo/2012-09-customer-experience-healthcare.pdf. Accessed December 11, 2012.

7. Bates S. Patient satisfaction in the age of social media. KevinMD.com. August 13, 2012; www.kevinmd.com/blog/2012/08/patient-satisfaction-age-social-media.html. Accessed November 14, 2012.

8. Schimpff S. Disruptive changes are coming to the delivery system. KevinMD.com. April 2, 2012; www.kevinmd.com/blog/2012/04/disruptive-coming-delivery-system.html. Accessed November 12, 2012.

9. Tehrani AB, Feldman SR, Camacho FT, Balkrishnan R. Patient satisfaction with outpatient medical care in the United States. *Health Outcomes Res Med.* 2011;2(4):e197-e202.

10. Salwitz J. My doctor is a computer! Sunrise Rounds Blog. April 10, 2012; http://sunriserounds.com/my-doctor-is-a-computer. Accessed November 14, 2012.

11. Dolan P. Physician rating website reveals formula for good reviews. amednews.com. February 27, 2012; www.ama-assn.org/amednews/2012/02/27/bil20227.htm. Accessed November 12, 2012.

12. Lagu T, Hannon NS, Rothberg MB, Lindenauer PK. Patients' evaluations of health care providers in the era of social networking: an analysis of physician-rating websites. *J Gen Intern Med.* 2010;25:942-946.

13. Goldman E. Doctors' Online Reputation Management and Patient Reviews. Technology & Marketing Law Blog. May 21, 2012; http://blog.ericgoldman.org/archives/2012/05/doctors_online.htm. Accessed November 14, 2012.

14. Lembke A. Why doctors prescribe opioids to known opioid abusers. *New Engl J Med.* 2012; 367:1580–1581.

15. Sepkowitz K. Doctor, Doctor, Give Me Reviews. Slate. November 28, 2008; www.slate.com/articles/health_and_science/medical_examiner/2008/11/doctor_doctor_give_me_reviews.html. Accessed November 8, 2012.

16. ElBoghdady D. Some doctors try to squelch online reviews. The WashingtonPost.com. January 28, 2012; http://articles.washingtonpost.com/2012-01-28/business/35441814_1_yelp-online-reviews-doctors/2.

17. Simons A. High court rules online posts didn't defame doctor. *Minneapolis Star Tribune.* January 30, 2013; http://www.startribune.com/local/189028521.html?refer=y. Accessed January 31, 2013.

18. Aleccia J. Toothache Lawsuit May Stifle Medical Gag Orders Against Online Rants. NBC News. November 30, 2011; http://vitals.nbcnews.com/_news/2011/11/30/9124107-toothache-lawsuit-may-stifle-medical-gag-orders-against-online-rants?lite. Accessed November 14, 2012.

19. Stewart EE, McMillen M. How to see your practice through your patients' eyes. *Fam Pract Manag.* 2008;15(6):18-20.

"A pessimist sees the difficulty in every opportunity; an optimist sees the opportunity in every difficulty."

—WINSTON CHURCHILL

CHAPTER 7

Professionalism in the Digital Age

UPDATING THE RULES OF PROFESSIONALISM

Several organizations and institutions have attempted to define a new aspect of professionalism specifically for social media. In the box on page 176, we've reprinted the official policy of the American Medical Association (AMA). These guidelines contain some good, commonsense advice regarding patient privacy and privacy of the physician's personal information on the Web. But the AMA document also contains several generalities such as "maintain appropriate boundaries of the patient-physician relationship in accordance with professional ethical guidelines" that could limit what doctors do in social media and does not go far enough in identifying what doctors *should* be doing with social media.

Data from state medical boards show that doctors have room for improvement when it comes to being professional online. A research letter published in the *Journal of the American Medical Association (JAMA)* in March 2012 detailed the results of a survey done to determine physician violations of online professionalism. Researchers surveyed 68 medical and osteopathic boards in all 50 states, the District of Columbia, and U.S. territories. Ninety-two percent reported at least one instance of an online professionalism violation, including inappropriate patient communication (i.e., sexual misconduct)—69%; prescribing online without an established clinical relationship—63%; and online misrepresentation of credentials—60%.[1]

Most of the boards also indicated that these infractions had been reported to them by patients, patients' families, and other medical professionals. Although the total number of incidents was small, the authors concluded that the frequency of occurrences could grow as the use of social media among physicians increases. This study underscores the need to create guidelines for physicians for appropriate online interactions due to the vastly greater visibility of social media.

AMA POLICY: PROFESSIONALISM IN THE USE OF SOCIAL MEDIA

The Internet has created the ability for medical students and physicians to communicate and share information quickly and to reach millions of people easily. Participating in social networking and other similar Internet opportunities can support physicians' personal expression, enable individual physicians to have a professional presence online, foster collegiality and camaraderie within the profession, provide opportunity to widely disseminate public health messages and other health communication. Social networks, blogs, and other forms of communication online also create new challenges to the patient-physician relationship. Physicians should weigh a number of considerations when maintaining a presence online:

(a) Physicians should be cognizant of standards of patient privacy and confidentiality that must be maintained in all environments, including online, and must refrain from posting identifiable patient information online.

(b) When using the Internet for social networking, physicians should use privacy settings to safeguard personal information and content to the extent possible, but should realize that privacy settings are not absolute and that once on the Internet, content is likely there permanently. Thus, physicians should routinely monitor their own Internet presence to ensure that the personal and professional information on their own sites and, to the extent possible, content posted about them by others, is accurate and appropriate.

(c) If they interact with patients on the Internet, physicians must maintain appropriate boundaries of the patient-physician relationship in accordance with professional ethical guidelines just, as they would in any other context.

(d) To maintain appropriate professional boundaries physicians should consider separating personal and professional content online.

(e) When physicians see content posted by colleagues that appears unprofessional they have a responsibility to bring that content to the attention of the individual, so that he or she can remove it and/or take other appropriate actions. If the behavior significantly violates professional norms and the individual does not take appropriate action to resolve the situation, the physician should report the matter to appropriate authorities.

(f) Physicians must recognize that actions online and content posted may negatively affect their reputations among patients and colleagues, may have consequences for their medical careers (particularly for physicians-in-training and medical students), and can undermine public trust in the medical profession.

Source: Copyright 1995-2013. American Medical Association. All Rights Reserved.

Another study, from the *Annals of Internal Medicine,* surveyed state medical boards, and asked them what kind of social media activity would prompt an investigation. Below are the results[2]:

- **High consensus** (Things more than three-quarters of the medical boards agreed would trigger an investigation):
  - Misleading claims on treatment outcomes or misrepresentation of board certification on a physician's website;
  - Posting photos of patients without their consent; and
  - Contacting a patient through an online dating site.
- **Moderate consensus** (Fewer than three-quarters but more than half of the medical boards said these would trigger an investigation):
  - Posting a photo on a social media site of doctor clearly intoxicated;
  - Posting patient narratives containing potential identifiers; and
  - Using discriminatory speech on a blog or social media site.
- **Low consensus** (Things that fewer than half of the medical boards said would trigger an investigation):
  - Posting something to a blog or social media site that is disrespectful of patients;
  - Posting patient narratives containing no potential identifiers; and
  - Posting a photo to a social media site that shows doctors drinking but not clearly intoxicated.

But online activity can also be a significant boost to a physician's reputation, enhance public trust in the profession, and lead to better health outcomes. Shouldn't the wide array of positive benefits to the profession also be considered? Professionalism in social media does not just encompass what *not to do;* it includes the imperatives of what we *must do* to maintain our professional image in this new era. Because social media has fundamentally changed the way all of us communicate and interact with others, it's difficult to imagine that we can continue to meet some of the professional commitments envisioned by the American Board of Internal Medicine (ABIM)—most notably the commitments to improving quality of care and access to care—without the help of social media tools. (See sidebar on pages 178–180.)

So how do you navigate the choppy waters of online reputation management and strengthen your reputation as an expert in your field and a caring physician while at the same time following all the protocols necessary for the utmost professionalism? You need a good social media profile. Following the guidelines in the previous chapters will put you well on your way to establishing a strong, positive digital footprint. As you do, you will need to be aware that social media has added a new dimension to the definition of professionalism. Here we'll give you some guidelines on using social media, both for professional and personal purposes.

MEDICAL PROFESSIONALISM IN THE NEW MILLENNIUM: A PHYSICIAN CHARTER

Principles of the Charter

The principles and responsibilities of medical professionalism must be clearly understood by both the profession and society. The three fundamental principles below are a guide to understanding physicians' professional responsibilities to individual patients and society as a whole.

Primacy of Patient Welfare

The principle is based on a dedication to serving the interest of the patient. Altruism contributes to the trust that is central to the physician-patient relationship. Market forces, societal pressures, and administrative exigencies must not compromise this principle.

Patient Autonomy

Physicians must have respect for patient autonomy. Physicians must be honest with their patients and empower them to make informed decisions about their treatment. Patients' decisions about their care must be paramount, as long as those decisions are in keeping with ethical practice and do not lead to demands for inappropriate care.

Social Justice

The medical profession must promote justice in the health care system, including the fair distribution of health care resources. Physicians should work actively to eliminate discrimination in health care, whether based on race, gender, socioeconomic status, ethnicity, religion, or any other social category.

Commitments of the Charter

The **Charter** commitments are a set of professional responsibilities that inform how physicians can practice the fundamental principles of the primacy of patient welfare, patient autonomy and social justice:

Commitment to professional competence.

Physicians must be committed to lifelong learning and be responsible for maintaining the medical knowledge and clinical and team skills necessary for the provision of quality health care. More broadly, the profession as a whole must strive to see that all of its members are competent and must ensure that appropriate mechanisms are available for physicians to accomplish this goal.

Commitment to honesty with patients.

Physicians must ensure that patients are completely and honestly informed before the patient has consented to treatment and after treatment has occurred. This expectation does not mean that patients should be involved in every minute decision about medical care; rather, they must be empowered

(Continued next page)

to decide on the course of therapy. Physicians should also acknowledge that in health care, medical errors that injure patients do sometimes occur. Whenever patients are injured as a consequence of medical care, patients should be informed promptly because failure to do so seriously compromises patient and societal trust. Reporting and analyzing medical mistakes provide the basis for appropriate prevention and improvement strategies and for appropriate compensation to injured parties.

Commitment to patient confidentiality.

Earning the trust and confidence of patients requires that appropriate confidentiality safeguards be applied to disclosure of patient information. This commitment extends to discussions with persons acting on a patient's behalf when obtaining the patient's own consent is not feasible. Fulfilling the commitment to confidentiality is more pressing now than ever before, given the widespread use of electronic information systems for compiling patient data such as electronic medical records (EMRs) and an increasing availability of genetic information. Physicians recognize, however, that their commitment to doctor-patient confidentiality must occasionally yield to overriding considerations in the public interest (for example, when patients endanger others).

Commitment to maintaining appropriate relations with patients.

Given the inherent vulnerability and dependency of patients, certain relationships between physicians and patients must be avoided. In particular, physicians should never exploit patients for any sexual advantage, personal financial gain, or other private purpose.

Commitment to improving quality of care.

Physicians must be dedicated to continuous improvement in quality health care. This commitment entails not only maintaining clinical competence but also working collaboratively with other professionals to reduce medical error, increase patient safety, minimize overuse of health care resources, and optimize the outcomes of care. Physicians must actively participate in the development of better measures of quality of care and the application of quality measures to assess routinely the performance of all health care professionals, institutions and systems. Physicians, both individually and through their professional associations, must take responsibility for assisting in the creation and implementation of mechanisms designed to encourage continuous improvement in the quality of care.

Commitment to improving access to care.

Medical professionalism demands that the objective of all health care systems be the availability of a uniform and adequate standard of care. Physicians must individually and collectively strive to reduce barriers to equitable health care. Within each system, the physician should work to eliminate barriers to access based on education, laws, finances, geography, and social discrimination. A

(Continued next page)

commitment to equity entails the promotion of public health and preventive medicine, as well as public advocacy on the part of each physician, without concern for the self-interest of the physician or the profession.

Commitment to a just distribution of finite resources.

While meeting the needs of individual patients, physicians are required to provide health care that is based on the wise and cost-effective management of limited clinical resources. They should be committed to working with other physicians, hospitals, and payers to develop guidelines for cost effective care. The physician's professional responsibility for appropriate allocation of resources requires scrupulous avoidance of superfluous tests and procedures. The provision of unnecessary services not only exposes one's patients to avoidable harm and expense but also diminishes the resources available for others.

Commitment to scientific knowledge.

Much of medicine's contract with society is based on the integrity and appropriate use of scientific knowledge and technology. Physicians have a duty to uphold scientific standards, to promote research, and to create new knowledge and ensure its appropriate use. The profession is responsible for the integrity of this knowledge, which is based on scientific evidence and physician experience.

Commitment to maintaining trust by managing conflicts of interest.

Medical professionals and their organizations have many opportunities to compromise their professional responsibilities by pursuing private gain or personal advantage. Such compromises are especially threatening in the pursuit of personal or organizational interactions with for-profit industries, including medical equipment manufacturers, insurance companies, and pharmaceutical firms. Physicians have an obligation to recognize, disclose to the general public, and deal with conflicts of interest that arise in the course of their professional duties and activities. Relationships between industry and opinion leaders should be disclosed, especially when the latter determine the criteria for conducting and reporting clinical trials, writing editorials or therapeutic guidelines, or serving as editors of scientific journals.

Commitment to professional responsibilities.

As members of a profession, physicians are expected to work collaboratively to maximize patient care, be respectful of one another, and participate in the processes of self-regulation, including remediation and discipline of members who have failed to meet professional standards. The profession should also define and organize the educational and standard-setting process for current and future members. Physicians have both individual and collective obligations to participate in these processes. These obligations include engaging in internal assessment and accepting external scrutiny of all aspects of their professional performance.

Reprinted with permission from The ABIM Foundation; The ACP Foundation, Copyright 2002.

A study of more than 4000 physicians conducted by Quantia in August 2011 showed that most were already involved in social media in some way; 67% said they used social media professionally, and 87% said they used it for personal reasons. A breakdown of use of some of the more popular sites showed that personal use is much higher than professional:

- YouTube: 8% professional; 31% personal;
- Facebook: 15% professional; 61% personal; and
- Twitter: 3% professional; 9% personal.

Nearly 90% of the doctors surveyed were not familiar with online patient communities, but two-thirds of those who were familiar with such sites said that the sites have a positive impact on patients. They found online patient communities to be especially useful for patients with rare diseases, cancer, and chronic conditions. Understandably, concerns about liability, privacy, time, and payment limit physicians from interacting with patients online.[3]

Influential social media leader Bryan Vartabedian, MD, a pediatric gastroenterologist in Texas, looks at a 2012 study in *Postgraduate Medical Journal*[4] and suggests that we change the inherent bias healthcare has against social media.

In the study "Influence of Social Networking Websites on Medical School and Residency Selection Process,"[4] investigators surveyed 600 U.S. medical school and residency admissions representatives regarding their use of social media profiles in the selection process.

Here are a few interesting stats:

- 9% report the use of social network profiles to evaluate applicants.
- 4% report having rejected an applicant based on social activity.
- 19% feel that it's a violation of privacy to search an applicant's social network activity.

Perhaps what the study does best is showcase medicine's entrenched cultural bias against social communication technology. Online professionalism is discussed here only in the context of the mischief that students can create rather than as an opportunity or obligation. Maybe we should recognize that many are doing good with these tools.

Here's an idea. Rather than choosing students based on their ability to master the standardized test, what about putting weight behind a "lifestream" or living e-portfolio of writing, curated material, recordings, and dialog that tell the real story of what drives an applicant? One application essay to understand an applicant? How about two years' worth of public essays? Instead of *avoiding* an applicant's public presence, the lifestream would represent a core determinant of candidacy for medical school.

Clearly we have a ways to go.

As long as we view publishing and communication technology from the perspective of risk rather than opportunity, the next generation of doctors will always be playing catch up.

Bryan Vartabedian, MD
Pediatric Gastroenterologist
Assistant Professor of Pediatrics
Baylor College of Medicine
Houston, Texas
http://33charts.com

GUIDE, INFORM, AND TEACH

Steering patients to worthwhile sources of information will become an important component of professionalism in medicine. A 2012 study in *The Journal of Pediatrics* looked at the accuracy of information on the Internet using a Google search pertaining to infant sleep safety. The authors started with 13 key phrases that a typical user might apply in searching for information on this subject. They then analyzed the first 100 websites for each phrase. They assessed the accuracy of the information based on how well it followed the recommendations of the American Academy of Pediatrics.[5]

The authors found that fewer than half (43.5%) of the 1300 websites studied offered accurate information on infant sleep safety. Another 28.1% gave inaccurate information, and 28.4% contained information that was not relevant. They also noted that government websites had the highest rate of accuracy and blogs the lowest. Even educational websites such as books, medical institution homepages, and peer-reviewed articles did not fare well in the study—only 52.4% of these sources contained accurate guidance. The authors acknowledged that some peer-reviewed articles were not available in their entirety because subscriptions are required, and that additional information might have been contained in the full article that would have affected the accuracy of the information found.[5]

By focusing on the kind of information patients find when they search the Web, this study underscores how much of the medical advice found there is not useful. Guiding patients to better online sources of medical information should be a new physician responsibility for the digital age. Not only should doctors expect and be receptive to questions patients raise from Web research, they need to proactively engage patients online in order to dispel falsehoods and guide them to legitimate sites.

Use social media to promote best practices of healthcare and medical developments that would interest the public. Many organizations and most medical journals use Twitter and other social media to post updates. By sharing their type of medical guidelines and advances with patients, we promote quality healthcare.

Don't feel like you have to update everyone on everything that's happening in the world of healthcare today. Choose subjects that interest you and topics that you find most relevant to your practice. It's much more productive to follow and write about issues that we're passionate about.

Respect copyright and intellectual property. You wouldn't plagiarize a colleague's work in print, so don't do it online either. Content curation is a valuable skill but link to the work of others or give attribution if you quote from other sources. Obtain permission from the owner of any photos, videos, or slide presentations you plan to use.

PROTECT YOURSELF WITH A SOCIAL MEDIA POLICY AND DISCLAIMER

If you run a medical practice, your employees are likely already engaging in social media. Many hospitals and medical organizations respond by blocking social media sites at work. At the 2012 Social Media Week conference at the Mayo Clinic, about half of the healthcare organizations represented said their institutions blocked social media.[6]

But employees today can still access Facebook and Twitter through their mobile phones. Rather than waste resources trying to stem that inevitable tide, it's more constructive to turn your employees into brand ambassadors, and teach them that they represent your practice and have to act responsibly online.

One way to do so is to implement a social media policy that describes the do's and don'ts of social media behavior. A sample list of policies from major health organizations is included in the Appendix. They have been constructed with great thought, so rather than starting from scratch, use them as a template to guide your own policy.

Simply having a policy isn't enough, however. Ensure that your employees have read and understood its contents.

Finally, it is a good idea to add a disclaimer to your own personal social media profiles if they are separate from those of your employer. Here's an example: "The opinions and statements on this site are my own and are not approved, reviewed, or endorsed by my employer or any other organization."

Explicitly state that you do not provide any personal medical advice and that you do not have a patient-physician relationship with your readers. Instruct readers to contact their own medical provider should they have any questions pertaining to their own health.

A HIGHER STANDARD THAN HIPAA

HIPAA is by now a well-known national standard for the protection of patient's health information. The Privacy Rule protects all "individually identifiable health information held or transmitted by a covered entity or its business associate, in any form or media, whether electronic, paper, or oral."[7]

Physicians must at all times guard against the disclosure of patient information. Consequently, responding to online reviews or engaging with a patient in an online conversation must be done with appropriate safeguards. Before you post anything online, whether it is on a review site, blog, or forum, remember that it is both public and permanent. Individual patient stories or case histories should never be posted online unless you have the patient's explicit consent. You don't really know who will ultimately read what you write online; so even if you believe you are contributing to a discussion that is not public, keep in mind that someone outside the medical profession may eventually read it.

HIPAA actually states that there are "no restrictions on the use or disclosure of de-identified health information." *But* the rule goes on to describe de-identified information as information that "neither identifies nor provides a reasonable basis to identify an individual." When you post information online, you are potentially reaching millions of people at one time. In this new age, it simply isn't possible to know for certain that no one will be able to identify the patient whose case you describe. Recall the story of the doctor in Rhode Island whose case was described in Chapter 3. This story is a cautionary tale of the consequences of posting any information about a single patient. The state medical board sanctioned this doctor, even though there was no HIPAA violation.

In the YouTube video "Digital Smarts," aimed at educating incoming medical interns, Vartabedian and pediatric resident Joey Spinner, MD, walk viewers through the following hypothetical Twitter update:

> I just saw the most amazing case of neonatal hemochromatosis . . . Not sure the little fella's going to make it.

This is technically HIPAA-compliant. But what if, they ask, that infant's mother happened to follow the doctor making that tweet and made the connection that it was her baby being discussed?

"I suspect that a lot of patients would have a problem with this," warns Vartabedian. "Potentially, this sort of ambient documentation represents a breach of trust. Call it a HIPAA-compliant breach of trust."[8]

Healthcare attorney David Harlow, an established blogger at Healthblawg.com, says that changing names and de-identifying patient information isn't enough.

"There are 18 elements that have to be stripped out of a story to have it considered de-identified under HIPAA. Number 18 is the tricky one—'anything else that can be used to re-identify the de-identified information,'" he says. "As more information is put online, it becomes harder and harder to say that this is something that couldn't be re-identified by someone else."[9]

When using social media, HIPAA cannot be the baseline for patient privacy in social media. Aim for a higher standard. Here are some other examples of unintended breaches of professionalism.

In 2009, a former neurosurgical resident from SUNY Upstate Medical University posted images from brain surgery on his Facebook profile.[10] The image was graphic, showing a man's head cut open and brain exposed. The pictures were visible to 260 of his friends, but not to the public. Here is a sample of some of the ensuing comments:

- "Do you feel like Hannibal Lector sometimes?"
- "Love a good BRAIN in the early morning!!"

It should be noted that no identifying information or connection to the medical school was present. After investigating, SUNY contacted the New York State Department of Health, and although no HIPAA violation was found, the physician was still reprimanded.

Another case surfaced a few months later at Stony Brook University Medical Center. In 2010, a photo of a medical student giving a "thumbs up" while posing with a cadaver during gross anatomy lab turned up on Facebook. The pictures belonged to a then emergency medicine resident, who had taken the images four years before. This unfortunate case made national headlines, and she was forced to publically apologize.[11] The one benefit from this particular case was that it spurred the medical school to formulate its social media policy.

As these examples demonstrate, you can't hide behind privacy settings. There is also no statute of limitations on inappropriate use. Every hospital needs a social media policy and should publicize it to their employees. It's better to know what's acceptable to post online beforehand, rather than deal with the aftereffects of a nationally publicized patient privacy breach.

Published stories of social media mishaps aren't going to endear doctors to using social media professionally, and that's a shame. But if we can use this as a valuable teaching point, rather than as a reason *not* to use social media, perhaps physicians can embrace it in a more responsible way rather than shunning it completely.

Katherine Chretien, MD, is an associate professor of medicine at George Washington University and one of the country's leading academic healthcare social media researchers. Here, she talks about how the bar of professionalism is raised when doctors are online:

> As someone who has been using social media for many years for both personal and professional use, as well as someone whose academic interest centers on online professionalism in medicine, I have great respect for the mark a physician's digital footprint leaves. Our words and actions online can carry such power—power to advocate, to educate, to connect, to reach, to transform, yet also the power to harm: others, patients, self, affiliated institutions, the profession. I try to remember that what I do online is an extension of my professional self so that the mark I leave is deliberate and what I intend.
>
> Why is online professionalism different from professionalism in our usual day-to-day lives as physicians? The core concepts are the same but there are some notable differences:
>
> 1. **Audience.** Online, there may be greater audiences involved, both intended and unintended. This works in physicians' favor when positive, professional messages are involved since they have greater reach and impact. This works against them when negative or unprofessional messages reach unintended audiences.
> 2. **Permanency.** Social media content is self-documenting and difficult to delete.
> 3. **Amplification.** Content can be amplified rapidly.
> 4. **Context.** Content can be misinterpreted more easily due to lack of accompanying context. Humor and sarcasm are particularly difficult to convey online.
>
> The concept of professionalism, though, evolves and depends heavily on cultural and social context. We have to be flexible enough to accommodate shifts in our standards based on changing social and generational norms while steadfast enough to uphold the stable tenets of ethics and

professionalism that are critical to public trust. How to strike this balance will be the challenge for medicine in the years to come.

Katherine Chretien, MD
Internal Medicine Physician
Associate Professor of Medicine
George Washington University
Washington, DC
www.mothersinmedicine.com

PROFESSIONALISM APPLIES TO PHYSICIAN-ONLY SITES TOO

What about physician-only social networks that are closed to the public, like Sermo or Doximity? Again, I would be careful here as well. There is no guarantee that posts will not leak out in the future. One need only look at a similar situation involving former *Washington Post* political blogger Dave Weigel.

Weigel covered the conservative movement for the *Post*, but also was involved with a progressive listserv called Journolist, which was closed to the public. On Journolist, progressive journalists, such as the *Washington Post's* Ezra Klein and the *New York Times'* Paul Krugman, would debate about, and sometimes savage, conservative politicians.

In 2010, some of Weigel's private Journolist posts were leaked, and they displayed a personal animosity to the conservatives that he was supposed to be objectively covering for the *Post*. The scandal forced him to resign from the newspaper.[12]

The lesson for health professionals is that what is private now may be publicized later. So even in private forums, maintain your professionalism.

COMMUNICATING WITH PATIENTS

With the healthcare-social media intersection being a relatively recent phenomenon, the thought of interacting with patients on social networks is giving some physicians pause. The study done by Quantia in 2011 found that 20% of the more than 4000 physicians it surveyed said they felt that any interaction with patients online is inappropriate.[3]

Many hospitals are also taking the approach that doctors are better off staying away from social media when it comes to connecting with patients. Ultimately, that's a losing strategy. Nuance is needed when it comes to the medical profession and social media. Just telling doctors to "stay away from patients on social media" is short-sighted.

Casting social media in a negative light will only stunt physician adoption of social media. While hospitals probably see this as a negligible tradeoff in order to protect their reputations, it's selfish and will make doctors even more tentative online. This puts them at a disadvantage at a time when patients expect more of their healthcare to involve the Web and social media.

A 2011 report by the research organization YouGov found that 81% of consumers believe that if a hospital has a strong social media presence, it is likely to be more cutting-edge, and 57% said that a social media connection with a hospital was likely to have a strong impact on their decision to seek treatment at that hospital.[13]

Utilizing social media properly gives physicians, and their affiliated hospitals, a powerful voice. Prominent physicians in the social space, like Vartabedian at Texas Children's Hospital, Wendy Sue Swanson, MD, at Seattle Children's Hospital, and Vineet Arora, MD, at the University of Chicago Medical Center, give their respective institutions a physician-branded credibility that's essential for trustworthiness online.

For now, social media hasn't evolved to a point where it can be used to provide personal medical advice to patients. But patients can still benefit from doctors active on social media. One way is by providing a physician's opinion on breaking medical news.

Every day, patients read health stories in the newspaper or watch them on television. And often, they are left with one simple question: "What do these stories mean to me?" Because of the 24-hour news cycle, health stories are often rushed and leave out precious physician commentary that gives patients proper context.

That's where social media comes in. Shortly after a story breaks, a doctor can write a blog post or go on Facebook or Twitter to share his or her professional opinion.

Consider cancer screening, for instance. Over the past few years, there have been controversy and changing guidelines on the way we screen for breast cancer and prostate cancer. The U.S. Preventive Services Task Force, an independent consortium of healthcare researchers that produces evidence-based practice guidelines, recently recommended against screening men for prostate cancer and questioned whether it was beneficial for younger women to undergo mammograms.[14]

These changing guidelines confuse patients. I regularly field calls from 65-year-old men asking whether they should have the prostate-specific antigen blood test to screen for prostate cancer, and from 40-year-old women asking whether a mammogram is appropriate for them.

A perspective piece from the *Journal of the National Cancer Institute* in 2011 crystallized the issue:

> There will come a time when all the patients have been followed, all the analyses done, all the groups assembled, and all the editorials written, and we still will not be secure in our knowledge of the individual harms and benefits of cancer screening. It appears that this time has come.[15]

If the medical profession is not secure in its knowledge of the risks and benefits of cancer screening, how can we expect patients to be?

I use my blog to talk about some of the under-reported issues that news stories ignore, such as the implications of a false-positive cancer screening test that can lead to further, more invasive tests that can harm patients. I also invite other primary care doctors and oncologists to provide their opinions in guest posts as well. This is the type of nuanced information that patients need in order to make a properly informed cancer screening decision.

Social media can be a powerful way for doctors to provide the meaning that patients crave when they read breaking health news in the media. A second way for doctors to engage patients with social media is to take the opportunity to educate them.

Pediatrician Swanson has a prominent social media presence, which includes her blog, Seattle Mama Doc, and on Twitter @SeattleMamaDoc. In a 2011 presentation at the Cerner Health Conference, she explains why doctors need to engage patients with social media[16]:

> We cannot just see our patients in the exam room. We need to be where people are. Clinicians need to experience using Twitter, Facebook and YouTube videos to interact with patients. Doctors also must be willing to share more of themselves to create a true partnership for better care . . . We have the great fortune to live in a time when we can communicate outside these walls.

And in the New York Times' Well blog, pediatrician Natasha Burgert, MD, describes how she uses social media to connect with adolescents. She reads teen blogs, and sometimes comments on them. In turn, her teenage patients read her blog as well as follow her on Twitter and Facebook. "I do as much as I can to get it on their phones, because that is what they live and die for," she says.[17]

Furthermore, in the exam room, instead of pamphlets and brochures on sexually transmitted diseases and safe sex practices that many teens may ignore, Burgert has a whiteboard filled with hyperlinks and QR codes. Teens can take a picture of the board with their smartphone and can read the material during their own time, in private.

What about patients who contact you online? It's not uncommon that I receive a message on Twitter or Facebook asking me to diagnose someone's abdominal pain or provide a second opinion for a set of tests.

Remember, it's OK to engage with patients collectively, but never individually on a social network. Offering personalized medical advice in the absence of an established doctor-patient relationship violates the rules of state medical boards and won't be covered by malpractice insurers.

I use a standard response in these cases, explaining that I cannot give personal medical advice on the Web, and then instruct these patients to contact their personal medical provider.

For established patients, I give another standard response, this time instructing them to call the office for an appointment or to dial 911 in case of an emergency. This takes the encounter offline, which is crucial since Twitter, Facebook, and blogs are public forums and not suitable for individualized doctor-patient dialogue. The final step is to briefly document the encounter in the patient's chart, as you would for a telephone conversation with a patient.

DON'T LET YOUR PERSONAL SOCIAL MEDIA LIFE DISTRACT YOU

Opinions vary widely on the topic of your personal online presence. Some experts believe that all personal use should be avoided. Internist Danielle Ofri, MD, wrote in the *New York Times* that she limits her online presence only to professional content.[18]

"This means letting go of the fun and casual side of social media, but I think that's simply part of the territory of being a doctor," she writes.

I don't think that's necessary. Instead, I recommend the dual citizenship approach that was previously discussed regarding Facebook in Chapter 4, whereby you maintain separate and distinct online profiles on social media sites. Physicians should be able to maintain their professional identity online and also have a private online identity to connect with family and friends.

But beware, the popularity of social media and proliferation of portable electronic devices such as smartphones, tablets, and the like are driving the attention of healthcare professionals away from patients. Think distracted driving is a problem? Try distracted doctoring.

Imagine that your neurosurgeon, during surgery, was talking on his or her cellphone using a headset. This unfortunate situation actually happened. A recent article in the *New York Times* cites a case where a patient was left paralyzed and the neurosurgeon was sued, in part, for being distracted. He made 10 personal calls during the operation. The article also cites a study from the journal *Perfusion* where 55% of technicians monitoring bypass machines admitted that they had made personal cell phone calls during heart surgery. Fifty percent had texted during surgery.[19]

We're encouraging more doctors to use "point of care" apps, which, in theory, should benefit patients. But unaccounted for is the fact that smartphones and tablets carry many other functions that are nonclinical—like Facebook, for instance.

"You walk around the hospital, and what you see is not funny," said Peter J. Papadakos, MD, an anesthesiologist and director of critical care at the University of Rochester Medical Center in upstate New York, who added that he has seen nurses, doctors, and other staff members glued to their phones, computers, and iPads.

"You justify carrying devices around the hospital to do medical records," he said. "But you can surf the Internet or do Facebook, and sometimes, for whatever reason, Facebook is more tempting."[19]

A simple answer, some say, would be to ban nonmedical use of smartphone and tablet apps. But like trying to ban texting and driving, that would be nearly impossible to enforce. A better approach would be increasing awareness and educating all healthcare professionals on the perils of such distractions.

SPECIAL CONSIDERATIONS FOR YOUNG PRACTITIONERS, RESIDENTS, AND STUDENTS

Issues with personal use of social media are more complicated for "digital natives." Most medical students and residents, and many young practitioners, have used digital technology from the time they were small children. It is as much a part of their everyday lives as television and newspapers are to people in an older generation. Most people under the age of 30 are accustomed to collaborating with peers over Facebook, playing multi-user games, texting frequently, and sharing information and files with friends and associates. But on my blog, medical students have commented that some academic medical centers are advising incoming medical residents to stay off social media. They have to close their blogs and shutter their Twitter or Facebook accounts.

From a hospital's standpoint, the damage that a single person can bring to an institution is considerable.

A study published in *JAMA* documented that a small minority (3%) of physician tweets were inappropriate,[20] while another paper found that 60% of medical schools reported that their medical students engaged in social media unprofessionally.

Violations included revealing patient information, depictions of intoxication, using discriminatory language, and posting sexually suggestive material.[21]

As hospitals and doctors try to use social media properly and prevent damage from its improper use, taking the extreme measure of forbidding doctors in training from using social media is heavy-handed and shortsighted, and, in the long run, will set doctors back in the increasingly influential online space.

Instead of an outright ban, academic institutions need to bring their culture into the 21st century, develop reasonable social media policies, and educate their staff. Social media cannot be framed as a threat, while the considerable benefits of appropriate physician social media use are ignored. Unfortunately, only 10% of medical schools have a social media policy.[22]

Social media should be part of the medical education curriculum. More digitally savvy physician role models are needed to teach residents and medical students not only how to act professionally online, but also how to harness their established social media knowledge as it applies to their future patients.

Shara Yurkiewicz is a medical student at Harvard Medical School, whose pieces have appeared in national publications such as the *Los Angeles Times*. Here she talks about the challenges she faces when writing patient stories online:

Storytelling is part of a physician's job. A doctor creates a narrative to communicate to a medical team. The prose is precise and the language is standardized, but the team wants to know what happens, in what order, what to do about it, and why.

The desire to share, however, sometimes extends beyond the confines of clinical care. During lunch, in the hallways, and in the elevators, my classmates and I trade snippets of what happened to our patients today. We know better, but we take the risk that even if strangers catch a few words here and there, not enough can be pieced together to violate confidentiality. It is part of the "hidden curriculum"—that is, being taught one thing in the classroom and practicing another in the workplace. None of this is new or news.

A major shift occurs when two things change: 1) the medium; and 2) the audience. We go online and write what we have previously shared in hushed tones over hospital meals. Our intentions are usually good: to share, to connect, to explain, to teach. But we are no longer looking our audience in the eye. We cannot see who our words reach, and we cannot see their effect. How do our responsibilities change?

I have found that the biggest challenge of writing as a medical student is the balance between confidentiality and honesty. During the first few days of medical school, I asked the higher-ups at my medical school for advice about boundaries in writing. Admitting it was a gray area that made heavy use of common sense, one of my advisers told me, "People aren't going to trust you enough to talk to you if they think you'll have no restraint in writing what they say. The classroom would no longer be a safe place."

Similarly, sometimes you meet a patient with an extraordinary story that you wish you could share, but it is too challenging to anonymize the details without losing the message. Here is where the specifics become even more confusing and peculiar. Sometimes I change identifying details (sex, age, location, temporality, or disease) or use a conglomeration of patients instead of just one. But doing this is inherently dishonest: even with a disclaimer, my story is partly fictional, and it is impossible to know which part. It becomes a representation of my perception rather than reality. If I want to make a specific point, what is stopping me from tweaking a detail or two to fit my worldview? Are my quotations verbatim, or are they close enough? Do I become a screenwriter rather than a physician if I change five details? Ten? Twenty?

Additionally, different rules surface depending on the outlet or story type. One major newspaper, for example, lets you omit details but not create them. It is also possible to seek the permission of the patient to tell a story. However, giving that person discretion over what smaller details are shared may change the story on a more macro level. It seems as though honesty and confidentiality lie on two opposing ends of a seesaw, but the audience is never sure which side is up.

As an employee of my hospital, I have access to every patient's online medical records. Each time I look up a patient, a box pops up. "Reason for looking up this patient?" My cursor hovers over the possible options: "Clinical care," "Teaching," "Research," "Admin," "Quality assurance"—it goes on. I instinctively head for the first or the second, because it's how I want to see myself. What I am doing is in the patient's best interest, or in my colleagues' best interest, or in the public's best interest.

But there is one option at the very end of the list that stands out: "Other." If you click "Other," you must explain why, on the record.

With online storytelling, I suspect there is a lot of "Other." But will we label it as such? Will we articulate why we need to share and who benefits from it? The rules are ambiguous enough today that I can push off the question, at least in medical records. It lingers in my mind though, as the details of what happens in Vegas slowly leak their way out.

Shara Yurkiewicz
Medical Student
Harvard Medical School
Brookline, Massachusetts
http://blogs.plos.org/thismayhurtabit

NAVIGATE THE ONLINE WATERS MINDFULLY

The Internet has fundamentally and permanently changed the doctor-patient relationship by breaking down the information walls traditionally separating patients from their healthcare professionals. How both parties navigate this new paradigm will determine how much the Web and social networks will positively impact healthcare.

Physicians should take advantage of these opportunities to educate patients, but also be perpetually aware of the consequences of our online activities. As social media evolves, the next big social network will always be around the corner. Friendster gave way to MySpace, which in turn gave way to Facebook. Who knows what's next? Guidelines tailored to individual sites cannot possibly keep up with the pace of social media innovation.

Always keep these general guidelines in mind whenever you're online. That way you can realize the potential of social media and know that your career won't be jeopardized while doing so. ⠿

REFERENCES

1. Greysen SR, Chretien KC, Kind T, Young A, Gross CP. Physician violations of online professionalism and disciplinary actions: a national survey of state medical boards. *JAMA*. 2012;307:1141-1142.

2. Greysen SR, Johnson D, Kind T, et al. Online professionalism investigations by state medical boards: first, do no harm. *Ann Intern Med*. 2013;158:124-130.

3. Modahl M, Tompsett L, Moorhead T. Doctors, Patients, and SocialMedia. QuantiaMD. 2011; www.quantiamd.com/q-qcp/DoctorsPatientSocialMedia.pdf. Accessed November 16, 2012.

4. Schulman CI, Kuchkarian FM, Withum KF, Boecker FS, Graygo JM. Influence of social networking websites on medical school and residency selection process. *Postgrad Med J*. 2012 Nov 8. [Epub ahead of print].

5. Chung M, Oden RP, Joyner BL, Sims A, Moon RY. Safe infant sleep recommendations on the Internet: let's Google it. *J Pediatr*. 20121;161:1080-1084.

6. Timimi F. HCAHPS Scores and Employee Social Media Access: Connected? Mayo Clinic Center for Social Media. October 19, 2012; http://socialmedia.mayoclinic.org/2012/10/19/hcahps-scores-and-employee-social-media-access-connected. Accessed November 16, 2012.

7. OCR. Department of Health and Human Services. Summary of the HIPAA Privacy Rule; www.hhs.gov/ocr/privacy/hipaa/understanding/summary/index.html. Accessed November 16, 2012.

8. Spinner J, Vartabedian B. Digital Smarts: A Common Sense Primer for Interns. YouTube. 2012; www.youtube.com/watch?v=hhNeIpVMdec&feature=share. Accessed November 16, 2012.

9. Healthcare Association of New York State. Health Care Social Media: Getting Executives on Board. April 2012; www.hanys.org/communications/social-media/assets/docs/health_care_social_media.pdf. Accessed November 1, 2012.

10. Mulder J. Posting of brain photo on Facebook sparks inquiry at Syracuse's Upstate Medical University. *Post Standard*. September 24, 2009; www.syracuse.com/news/index.ssf/2009/09/posting_of_brain_photo_on_face.html. Accessed November 16, 2012.

11. Einiger J. Facebook Cadaver Photo Comes Back to Haunt Stony Brook University Medical Center Student. 7online.com. WABC TV. February 2, 2010; http://abclocal.go.com/wabc/story?section=news/local&id=7253275. Accessed November 16, 2012.

12. Triplett M. WaPo's Dave Weigel Resigns After More Journolist E-Mails Surface. Mediaite. June 25, 2010; www.mediaite.com/online/wapos-dave-weigel-resigns-after-more-journolist-e-mails-surface. Accessed November 16, 2012.

13. Consumers' Use, Preferences, and Expectations of Hospital Social Media. YouGov, PLC. November 1, 2011.

14. Screening for Prostate Cancer. Topic Page. U.S. Preventive Services Task Force. May 2012; www.uspreventiveservicestaskforce.org/prostatecancerscreening.htm. Accessed November 16, 2012.

15. Stefanek ME. Uninformed compliance or informed choice? A needed shift in our approach to cancer screening. *J Natl Cancer Inst*. 2011;103:1821-1826.

16. CHC 2011 General Session Recap: Dr. Wendy Sue Swanson. Cerner.com. October 11, 2011; www.cerner.com/blog/chc_2011_general_session_recap_dr_wendy_sue_swanson. Accessed November 16, 2012.

17. Hoffman J. Texting the Teenage Patient. New York Times Well Blog. October 8, 2012; http://well.blogs.nytimes.com/2012/10/08/texting-the-teenage-patient. Accessed November 6, 2012.

18. Ofri D. Should Your Doctor Be on Facebook? New York Times Well Blog. April 28, 2011; http://well.blogs.nytimes.com/2011/04/28/should-your-doctor-be-on-facebook/?partner=rss&emc=rss. Accessed November 18, 2012.

19. Richtel M. As doctors use more devices, potential for distraction grows. *New York Times*. December 15, 2011; www.nytimes.com/2011/12/15/health/as-doctors-use-more-devices-potential-for-distraction-grows.html?pagewanted=all&_r=0. Accessed November 16, 2012.

20. Chretien KC, Azar J, Kind T. Physicians on Twitter. *JAMA*. 2011;305:566-568.

21. Chretien KC, Greysen SR, Chretien J-P, Kind T. Online posting of unprofessional content by medical students. *JAMA*. 2009;302:1309–1315.

22. Kind T, Genrich G, Sodhi A, Chretien KC. Social media policies at US medical schools. *Med Educ Online*. 2010;15: doi: 10.3402/meo.v15i0.5324.

"Never doubt that a small group of committed people can change the world. Indeed it is the only thing that ever has."

—Margaret Mead

CHAPTER 8

Connect and Be Heard: My Journey from Social to Mainstream Media

Anyone passionate about social media will tell you that it is very frustrating when peers don't understand the value of this technology. However, this is also a great opportunity to educate. I realized early on that social media is the best way to take control of my digital footprint. There is a natural fear surrounding social media and a common misconception that it is all fluff and not something that you can afford to invest time in.

One day, I was talking to a colleague about how social media had the potential to fundamentally change the professional lives of doctors. I shared some stories that I had witnessed surrounding social media, many of which are included in previous chapters of this book. Still, this person was not convinced, and he remained skeptical.

"I see 25 patients a day, return phone calls, do insurance paperwork, and then make rounds in the hospital," he said. "Who has time for social media? I don't see how it's going to make a difference."

I can confidently say that social media has certainly made a difference in my life. It has opened up many professional doors for me, opportunities that I couldn't have dreamed of while training in medical school and residency. I believe that my journey with social media has not only made a difference in my own life, but that it can also make a difference and improve the current healthcare system as we know it.

IT ALL STARTS WITH YOU

I started to engage with patients online in the early 2000s, a few years before I started my blog. At that time, we were all watching Google begin its meteoric rise.

The search-based website had just introduced a little-known service called Google Answers. This was a site where anyone could ask a question, and a team of highly trained Google Answers researchers would search the Web and provide answers. When I took a closer look at the site, some of those questions were health-related, and it was a bit disturbing to me that people without a healthcare background were answering these questions.

I saw an opportunity and applied to become a Google Answers researcher. The entire process was slightly less rigorous than applying to medical school . . . but I forged ahead. Google put me through a series of obscure search tasks, so you can imagine how excited I was when I received an e-mail from Google proclaiming that I was accepted as a Google Answers researcher.

I was eager to contribute and immediately started answering patient questions. At first, the questions were general:

- "What are the side effects of this medication?"
- "What are some potential complications of this surgical procedure?"

However, over time the questions started becoming more personal.

- "What could be causing my abdominal pain?"
- "Can you give a second opinion on my husband's cancer diagnosis?"

THE TIME WAS CHANGING

Someone even uploaded a copy of lab tests for me to interpret. This was indeed a different time period, where all of this technology and interaction were brand new. It was before social media guidelines, and before I had the knowledge and insight to realize that that by answering these questions I was potentially putting my professional career in jeopardy.

Some people discovered my e-mail address and started e-mailing me health questions to answer. Some uploaded high-resolution images of every body part imaginable. I'll leave it to your imagination as to what some of those body parts were.

One evening I was staring at my inbox full of questions from patients that I didn't even know, and I realized that patients were no longer getting the information they needed only in the doctor's office. It was an indictment of the doctor-patient relationship as we knew it.

It was at that moment that I also realized how vital the Internet would be in bridging that information void.

Previous chapters of this book have covered how social media can connect healthcare professionals with not only their patients, but also their colleagues. However, social media can be taken one step further, even beyond defining your reputation online. It can give you a voice and a platform to communicate and allow you to be heard in the national healthcare conversation.

CRASH COURSE IN HEALTH POLICY

On KevinMD.com, I regularly publish guest posts—not only from other doctors but also from other players in the healthcare arena such as nurses, medical students, patients, and even lawyers.

A few years ago, I invited a plaintiff attorney to write a guest article on medical malpractice. This is an issue about which, for the most part, physicians have a fairly unified view. When this attorney's post was published, it generated a firestorm of comments—not only from doctors, but from other lawyers and injured patients as well.[1]

One particular comment from a patient caught my attention. He wrote that "KevinMD.com is the only site on the web where you could get doctors, lawyers and patients all together in one place debating a contentious issue like medical malpractice in a relatively civilized and constructive manner."

That moment is when it dawned on me that social media could offer a powerful forum for debate.

Debate is important because there are very few healthcare issues that everyone agrees upon. Consider the healthcare reform environment, which currently engages the United States. There are very few topics that are considered more polarizing.

However, I strongly believe that people can learn from the opposition. With that in mind, I encourage a variety of viewpoints that cross the political spectrum on KevinMD.com. I personally have learned a tremendous amount from reading the competing healthcare visions from the progressive and conservative points of view.

THE TRADITIONAL MAINSTREAM MEDIA ARE CALLING

That knowledge and insight gained from reading guest articles on my blog came in handy when an editor from the *New York Times* contacted me early in 2009.

"Dr. Pho," she wrote in an e-mail, "would you like to contribute a piece to Room for Debate?"

Room for Debate was a blog on the *New York Times'* website where outside experts from various fields engaged in a spirited debate by writing short opinion pieces. The topic for this occasion was healthcare reform. The editor asked if I would write a health policy piece commenting on what President Obama said during his State of the Union address.

As a primary care doctor, I realized that I did not have any health policy training whatsoever and thought to myself that there was no way I could possibly contribute. However, when I expressed these concerns, the editor replied, "Try your best. We want to hear from the perspective of a practicing physician."

So after watching the President's speech, I sat down and began writing my commentary. As I wrote, I discovered that the task was easier than I had anticipated. I realized that I had learned a tremendous amount about health policy already—not from a formal classroom setting but from my blog and other forms of social media.

Reading the perspectives from the guest authors on KevinMD.com, combined with the articles recommended by the health policy thought leaders that I had followed on Twitter, gave me more than enough background information to write the *New York Times'* commentary.

OPENING THE SOCIAL DOORS

When my piece was published on the website the next day, I was shocked. Above my piece was an article from Elliot Fisher, MD, MPH, professor of medicine at Dartmouth University School of Medicine. He is a well-known public policy speaker and is frequently cited in major mainstream media outlets. Also featured was an article from Daniel Callahan, PhD, founder of the Hastings Center, a prominent, nonpartisan public policy institute.

And on the very same page, there was my commentary.[2] At the time, this was an astounding accomplishment for a doctor who literally learned everything he knew about health policy from reading blogs and following thought leaders on Twitter.

Now, I'm not saying that I'm anywhere near the level of those health policy luminaries. But just the fact that I shared a major medium platform with them was nothing short of amazing.

Social media has not only given me a basic health policy education, it has also given me the opportunity to share my opinion in the *New York Times*, as well as in major media channels like *USA Today*, CNN, and Fox News, where I've written columns on health policy entities like Accountable Care Organizations and Patient-Centered Medical Homes.

My journey with the media has also led me to Washington, DC. On July 17, 2009, I participated in a panel discussion at the National Press Club, discussing and debating health policy with other experts. It was a tremendous opportunity for a practicing primary care physician like myself to have my voice heard in the heart of the health-care reform movement.

Social media not only gave me my health policy voice, it also gave me the opportunity to have that voice heard.

THE HUMANIZATION OF MEDICAL PROFESSIONALS

Getting your voice heard also helps in another area—public relations. Just as doctors have little training in health policy during medical school and residency, they have zero education in public relations and engaging the media. That fact contributes to the sinking reputation of many doctors today.

In the documentary "The Vanishing Oath," directed by emergency physician Ryan Flesher, MD, individuals on the streets of Boston were interviewed by his producer, Nancy Pando, about what they thought about doctors. Here are some of their responses[3]:

> **Nancy Pando:** Why do you think someone chooses to become a doctor?
>
> **Interviewee #1:** That's definitely a job you take on because you want to do it, not because you want to make money. And a lot of [doctors] don't do it for the right reasons.
>
> **Pando:** And a lot of them do it, why?
>
> **Interviewee #1:** Just to make money . . . and to have clout so they can go to these big galas and fundraisers to talk about all the great things they can do, but not actually do them.
>
> **Interviewee #2:** In my experience, more doctors than not are out just to make money. I would say that if you took five doctors, four are out to make money. And one of them cares.
>
> **Pando:** Would you say that most doctors are looking at the dollars and cents?
>
> **Interviewee #3:** Absolutely.

Unfortunately, these three interviewees are not alone in thinking this way. When I wrote a piece in *USA Today* on chronic pain management, a letter to the editor published in reply said, in part, "Doctors prescribe drugs so that they can get to the golf course a little bit earlier."[4]

That perception that doctors are in it for the money, or that they prescribe drugs so that they can have more leisure time, quite frankly is a slap in the face to the medical profession. I take statements like those personally, which slight the majority of doctors who aren't in it for the money or who go that extra mile for their patients.

Consider this description of a typical day that internist Danielle Ofri, MD, posted in a New York Times Well Blog article[5]:

> I would get up at the crack of dawn to round on the hospitalized patients, then rush to the office for a full slate of scheduled patients. Throughout the day, I'd field calls from the nurses in the hospital: Someone's potassium was low. A patient had new symptoms of nausea. A feeding tube was clogged. The M.R.I. results were back. Dialysis was canceled. It was the worst feeling in the world, trying to focus on patients in the office while managing my hospitalized patients by phone until I could finish up, then racing back to the hospital for evening rounds. I knew I was doing a substandard job with both sets of patients, but I couldn't be in two places at once. This was simply unsustainable.

Or consider this timeline of a typical morning of pediatrician Heather MacAdam, MD, written in a U.S. News and World Report blog[6]:

> **6:00 a.m.**—Alarm rings—hit snooze. Today I have nursery rounds, so I slap on some scrubs and head out the door to the hospital. I gave up wearing nice clothes to work after being vomited on one too many times during training.

> **7:00 a.m.**—Newborn nursery rounds. The nurses line the babies up one by one to be seen. Nothing wakes you up like a line of screeching babies waiting for you. After checking their weight and vital signs, I wheel them back to their mothers and offer advice and congratulations.

> **8:00 a.m.**—Head to the practice. Today is fully booked—as I walk in, I notice a waiting room full of playing children and can't help but wonder what germs they might be passing to each other.

> **8:00 a.m.–12:00 p.m.**—Pediatric appointments. The clinic schedules each child for a 15-minute appointment—regardless of the complexity of the problem. As usual, I'm running 30 minutes behind, trying to catch up with the inevitable and unplanned surprises that pop up. The new electronic medical records we are using are nice for some things, but it takes me twice as long to document a visit.

CHANGING PUBLIC PERCEPTION ONE BLOG, TWEET, AND STATUS UPDATE AT A TIME

These are the stories that all medical professionals have versions of and that must be told via social media to humanize our profession. We need to let the public know that doctors are caring humans, mothers and fathers, brothers and sisters, and sons and daughters. We need to share the stories of the sacrifices every healthcare professional makes to function in a system that stacks the deck against good patient care.

Sometimes, changing the public perception requires doctors to provide another side to commonly reported issues. Take medical malpractice, for example. Thankfully, I've never been sued for medical malpractice. However, that puts me in the minority, as 61% of doctors will get sued sometime during their careers.[7]

Much of the focus when it comes to medical malpractice is on the contention between doctors and lawyers, and sometimes the voice of the injured patient is heard. But has anyone thought about the doctor who has been accused of malpractice? Whenever I bring this issue up to my non-physician friends, I'm met with a lack of sympathy. "Who cares about that physician," they say. "Isn't he or she the one who made the mistake?"

This is not always necessarily true. A well-cited 1999 Institute of Medicine report showed that 100,000 patient deaths a year were due to medical mistakes, but a closer look found that 90% of these mistakes weren't due to negligent physicians, but to systems errors in our medical institutions.[8] When a doctor gets sued, it's an emotionally traumatic experience. *American Medical News* interviewed some of these physicians, and here is what they had to say[9]:

"Being sued is a life altering experience."

"Surviving a lawsuit is like overcoming a death."

"The impact of a medical malpractice trial could last a lifetime."

"You go through a phase where you question everything. You really question your worth as a doctor."

Being sued is associated with burnout, depression, and an increased risk of suicide, all of which make these doctors more prone to future medical mistakes. That is an important statement, since many physicians who have been sued will continue to practice medicine.

We need to use social media to share this view on malpractice—a view patients most likely are not informed about. It's important for the public to hear about this issue from a physician's perspective because medical malpractice affects not only doctors, but also the care patients receive.

This is exactly what emergency physician Edwin Leap, MD, sets out to do with his blog. An eloquent writer, Leap paints a powerful picture of how medical malpractice impacts doctors. This quote from his blog showcases his powerful writing[10]:

For many physicians, medicine is the single most important validation of their lives. Doctor, physician, healer, professional . . . are the words that come to mind. Malpractice, however, replaces them with assailant, defendant, killer, and quack. Malpractice takes that validation and shatters it into a million pieces. Threatening loss of work, loss of money and livelihood, loss of reputation, it ends in loss of self-image and loss of self-worth. And for all too many physicians, that loss compounds the other stresses of practice, and makes death seem a reasonable, even desirable, alternative.

These are the stories that put a human face on doctors and are a powerful way that we can change the public perception of the medical profession.

FROM SOCIAL TO MAINSTREAM MEDIA

In a review of my site, blogger David Catron wrote that "a comment stream on one of KevinMD's posts provides more insight than any other source can ever hope to impart."[11] Those words crystallize exactly what I try to do—pull back the curtain and allow patients a peek at the behind-the-scenes world of healthcare.

This process is important because healthcare professionals should have more involvement with and influence on politicians in Washington. An excellent way to get through to politicians on both sides of the aisle is via their constituents—our patients. So it's imperative that we let the public know that the more difficult it is to practice medicine, the harder it is to give patients the care that they deserve and demand.

BE READY FOR AN OPPORTUNITY

Social media allows real-world physicians to share their stories from behind the scenes, which can lead to amazing opportunities. In October 2007, "CBS Evening News" did a story entitled "Defensive Medicine: Cautious Or Costly?"[12] The segment told the story of college student Alexandra Varipapa who went to the emergency department because of abdominal pain. There she underwent a costly CT scan, and her father—a physician—argued that a less expensive pelvic exam and ultrasound should have been performed instead. He claimed that the hospital practiced defensive medicine.

A few months before the story, "CBS Evening News" came to Nashua, New Hampshire, transformed my small office into a temporary television studio, and interviewed me for the piece. The following is an excerpt of that the interview that made it on air[12]:

> Dr. Kevin Pho runs the popular medical blog KevinMD, where doctors routinely confess exactly how they run up costs by practicing defensive medicine.

> "Defensive medicine is bad medicine," Pho said.

In a post, one ER doctor says he's just admitted two patients to the hospital—when he was sure "neither was having cardiac (problems), but what am I to do?"

Another admits that in his practice, "every patient with a headache gets a (CT) scan."

"It's much easier to defend the fact that you ordered a test than it is to not order the test at all," Pho said.

And the costs of defensive medicine today are increasingly paid by patients, even those with insurance because of rising deductibles and co-payments.

"There's no doubt in my mind this is a significant driver in healthcare costs today," Pho said.

Out of all the physicians in the country that "CBS Evening News" could have chosen for this story, it chose me—a relatively anonymous private practice physician in southern New Hampshire. What set me apart from the rest is simple. My blog and my ease and availability to be contacted were the reasons I was selected. In 2007, not many doctors were exploring social media. An additional benefit of the experience was that the physician voices on my blog were elevated to a national television platform in the "CBS Evening News" story.

JOIN THE CONVERSATION

I have traveled the country speaking with doctors about social media and online reputation, and the topic of healthcare reform invariably comes up. It is apparent that many physicians feel despair and helplessness surrounding the world of new media and medicine. "I know the way we're going to practice medicine is going to change," said one doctor. "But I feel there's not a damn thing I can do about it."

I disagree with some of my colleagues' views on this subject. There is a strong and important group that is interested in what we have to say: our patients.

A 2009 Gallup survey asked a sample of U.S. citizens who they trusted the most when it came to health reform: the President, Congress, health policy experts, or doctors. Shocking to some of the industry, doctors came in first place.[13]

Patients still trust doctors, and they want to hear what we have to say. That's why I advise healthcare professionals that, no matter their political stripes, they need to share their opinion on healthcare reform and get involved in the conversation.

Sometimes, that requires a bigger stage than social media can provide. It means going on television, doing radio interviews, and writing columns and op-eds for newspapers. As a member of the Board of Contributors for *USA Today*, I have the fortunate opportunity to discuss major healthcare issues that I think need to be better articulated on the national stage, such as:

+ The lack of primary care doctors;
+ The fact that our emergency departments are growing more crowded; and
+ The fact that more of our doctors and nurses are suffering career burnout.

NO TRAINING REQUIRED

If I am able to utilize social media, then so can every doctor, every nurse, and every healthcare professional. Before starting my journey I didn't have any media training in medical school or residency. I didn't take any public relations courses. I didn't even write for my school newspaper. I learned to write an op-ed piece by Googling "how to write an op-ed."

I realized that the skills that I had been building while communicating in social media since 2004 gave me some of the tools necessary to connect with the mainstream media. I wrote blog posts every day, which polished my writing skills and gave me the confidence to submit pieces that got accepted by national publications. I recorded online podcasts, which helped prepare me for my first live radio interview. Finally, there is no better way to practice for a television appearance than doing patient education videos on YouTube.

I currently talk to the media several times a week, and it's a tremendous opportunity to give a physician's perspective on breaking health news, provide commentary on healthcare reform, or even explain why more healthcare professionals need to be involved with social media.

Reporters often reach out to physicians on social media, finding them to be an accessible, authoritative source of medical opinion. In 2011, the Oriella PR Network studied journalist usage of social media. Forty-seven percent of journalists said they used Twitter for new story ideas, 35% said they used Facebook, and 30% used blogs that they were familiar with.[14] I field numerous reporter queries weekly just from the visibility I have on my blog or on Twitter.

For healthcare professionals interested in amplifying their voice using mainstream media, here are a few tips that I've learned along the way:

+ **Be available.** Make sure that your contact information is accessible from your social media platforms. For instance, include a "Contact me" page on your blog, which contains your e-mail address, or a form that can be sent to you. I've seen too many physician blogs where there is no way to contact the author.
+ **Be responsive.** When a reporter or television producer contacts you, it is often because of a breaking story, and he or she is under a time deadline. If you want to

be quoted or contribute to an article, you'll have to respond quickly. Otherwise, the person will move on to another expert.

- **Be concise.** Make your points in sound-bite-size pieces. Whether talking to a newspaper reporter or doing a live television interview, your contribution will have much more impact if you package your answers in quotable sound bites.

- **Be experienced.** While you can cite numbers and statistics during your media appearance, an added anecdote can make your argument connect with the public. Draw from your clinical experience, in a HIPAA-compliant fashion of course, to paint a vivid picture and get your point across.

- **Be promotional.** Engaging with the media is a tremendous way to not only spread your influence, but also to enhance your reputation. Reporters, along with radio and television producers, will ask how you would like to be cited. Depending on your situation, you can include your practice, blog, or social media presence. Politely ask reporters to link to your website in the online version of their story. This will not only bring you a traffic boost, but links from newspaper websites are valuable in the eyes of Google and can help with search engine optimization.

- **Be prepared.** Allow yourself to be open for future opportunities. Once you've gained a mainstream media audience, other outlets will call. The dynamic nature of breaking health news, combined with the contention that surrounds healthcare reform, means that the public wants to hear what physicians and other healthcare professionals think. Use your growing media presence to increase that transparency between doctors and patients.

LEARN FROM OTHERS IN OUR FIELD

I'm not the only doctor who has made the jump from social to mainstream media. Here are three others:

- Mike Sevilla, MD, a family physician in Ohio, has both a blog and an online podcast where he discusses current health issues and advocates for the importance of the family doctor. His social media activity created the opportunity to appear on his local television news, where he was interviewed in a health segment. After several more appearances, he's now a regular contributor.

- Wendy Sue Swanson, MD, is a pediatrician in Seattle. In addition to her blog, she produces regular YouTube videos where she draws upon her own experiences as a parent to help educate her patients and their families. She also has commented on national news stories and appears regularly on her local television news program.

- Natasha Burgert, MD, is a pediatrician in Kansas City. She was featured in a *New York Times* article on digital doctors, chronicling how she used social media and texting to educate her teen patients.[15] That garnered the attention of "CBS This Morning," which gave her the opportunity to fly to New York City and be interviewed on national television. The exposure made her a prominent example of how doctors can successfully incorporate digital technology into their practice.

The four of us have social media to thank for providing the opportunities to connect with mainstream media. These media skills are critical for every healthcare professional to have if we hope to have a say in the changing healthcare world around us.

MAKE A DIFFERENCE IN HEALTHCARE

I've been involved with the healthcare/social media intersection almost since the beginning, and I've seen it change and impact lives in ways both good and bad. Like the powerful waves of the ocean, social media's viral and public nature must be respected. I've watched the careers of promising young physicians get derailed because of social media. I've seen a doctor forced to settle a medical malpractice suit simply because of his blog. I have witnessed hospitals having to deal with embarrassing national headlines because of inappropriate use of social media.

It would be one-sided to ignore the risks involved when healthcare professionals use social media. However, if we're too paralyzed by fear to take these risks, how can we realize the tremendous potential social media has in healthcare?

The potential to give patients a voice in their care outweighs any risk. The potential to connect clinicians from around the world so that they can learn from and teach each other outweighs any risks. Finally, for me personally, the potential to give every healthcare professional a way to enter the national healthcare conversation and be heard outweighs any risks.

In fact, the biggest risk of social media in healthcare is not using it at all.

Despite what I've seen, the healthcare social media journey is just beginning. Our industry is still trying to find ways to incorporate social media's value into the lives of patients, doctors, and hospitals.

How quickly that happens depends on you. After reading this book, hopefully you'll be convinced of social media's power to define your online reputation, connect with patients and colleagues, make your voice heard, and help educate the patient population. As a healthcare professional, you not only need to convince your colleagues of social media's value, but guide them on their social media journeys as well.

When we look at the big picture, that is a tremendous responsibility. However, it's a responsibility we must embrace; it's an opportunity we cannot miss.

Social media has already changed the world, and with your help it can create a better, open, transparent, and honest healthcare system for all. ⊞

REFERENCES

1. Nash B. Open dialogue on medical malpractice. KevinMD.com. 2010; www.kevinmd.com/blog/2010/12/open-dialogue-medical-malpractice-patient-safety.html.

2. Editors. Ideas for Fixing Health Care. *New York Times*. February 25, 2009; http://roomfordebate.blogs.nytimes.com/2009/02/25/ideas-for-fixing-health-care. Accessed November 6, 2012.

3. Crash Cart Productions. The Vanishing Oath; www.crashcartproductions.com. Accessed November 6, 2012.

4. Letters: Doctors Can't Grant Every Wish. *USA Today*. September 28, 2011; http://usatoday30.usatoday.com/news/opinion/letters/story/2011-09-28/hospitals-patient-satisfaction-surveys/50594286/1. Accessed November 6, 2012.

5. Ofri D. The Ins and Outs of the Doctor's Day. New York Times Well Blog. June 7, 2012; http://well.blogs.nytimes.com/2012/06/07/the-ins-and-outs-of-the-doctors-day. Accessed November 6, 2012.

6. Medical School Admissions Doctor. Follow a Day in the Life of a Primary Care Physician. U.S.News.com; November 7, 2011; www.usnews.com/education/blogs/medical-school-admissions-doctor/2011/11/07/follow-a-day-in-the-life-of-a-primary-care-physician. Accessed November 6, 2012.

7. Krupa C. Medical liability: by late career, 61% of doctors have been sued. amednews.com. August 16, 2010; www.ama-assn.org/amednews/2010/08/16/prl20816.htm. Accessed November 6, 2012.

8. Kohn LT, Corrigan JM, Donaldson M. *To Err Is Human: Building a Safer Healthcare System*. Washington, DC: National Academies Press; 1999.

9. Gallegos A. Life after lawsuit: how doctors pick up the pieces. amednews.com. May 16, 2011; www.ama-assn.org/amednews/2011/05/16/prsa0516.htm. Accessed November 6, 2012.

10. Leap E. Malpractice and Suicide (July EMN column). Edwinleap.com. 2007; http://edwinleap.com/blog/?p=67. Accessed November 6, 2012.

11. Catron D. A post about a post about a blogger. Health Care BS. August 18, 2007; www.healthcarebs.com/2007/08/18/a-post-about-a-post-about-a-blogger. Accessed November 6, 2012.

12. Defensive Medicine: Cautious or Costly? CBS News. October 22, 2007; www.cbsnews.com/stories/2007/10/22/eveningnews/main3394654.shtml. Accessed November 6, 2012.

13. Saad L. On Healthcare, Americans Trust Physicians Over Politicians. Gallop Politics. June 17, 2009; www.gallup.com/poll/120890/healthcare-americans-trust-physicians-politicians.aspx. Accessed November 6, 2012.

14. Latta S. Social Media Infiltrates the Newsroom and Optimism Returns to Journalism According to Fourth Annual Oriella Study. HORN. Blog. May 18, 2011; www.horngroup.com/#/blog/social-media-infiltrates-the-newsroom-and-optimism-returns-to-journalism-according-to-fourth-annual-oriella-study. Accessed November 6, 2012.

15. Hoffman J. Texting the Teenage Patient. New York Times Well Blog. October 8, 2012; http://well.blogs.nytimes.com/2012/10/08/texting-the-teenage-patient. Accessed November 6, 2012.

Appendix

RECOMMENDED BLOGS

Bryan Vartabedian, MD: 33 Charts
http://33charts.com

Christopher Johnson, MD
www.chrisjohnsonmd.com/blog

Claire McCarthy, MD: MD Mama
www.boston.com/lifestyle/health/mdmama

iMedicalApps.com
www.imedicalapps.com

Jordan Grumet, MD: In My Humble Opinion
http://jordan-inmyhumbleopinion.blogspot.com

Karen Sibert, MD: A Penned Point
http://apennedpoint.com

Rob Lamberts, MD: Musings of a Distractible Mind
http://more-distractible.org

Robert Wachter, MD: Wachter's World
http://community.the-hospitalist.org

Suzanne Koven, MD: In Practice
www.boston.com/lifestyle/health/blog/inpractice

Wendy Sue Swanson, MD: Seattle Mama Doc Blog
http://seattlemamadoc.seattlechildrens.org

KEVIN PHO'S CURATED TWITTER LIST

http://twitter.com/kevinmd/essential

SUGGESTED SOCIAL MEDIA READING

Bryan Vartabedian, MD: Physicians, Risk and Opportunity in the Digital Age (http://goo.gl/Kiei5)

 This long post is based on a Pediatric Grand Rounds that Dr. Vartabedian delivered at Texas Children's Hospital on December 2, 2011. It can serve as a handy guide on social media in healthcare and how it's redefining the role of the physician. Vartabedian addresses "some of the challenges that physicians face including transparency, boundaries of the doctor/patient relationship and the moral obligation to participate." He presents a balanced discussion of the opportunities and risks that social media presents.

Bryan Vartabedian, MD: The Case for New Physician Literacies in the Digital Age (http://goo.gl/TYva3)

 This post is based on a presentation given by Dr. Vartabedian at Stanford's Medicine X on September 30, 2012. It focuses on how the transformation of information in the digital age is changing the way doctors get and use information in their medical practices. He includes key literacies—"broad skill sets needed to function"—that are important for physicians today.

Healthcare Association of New York State: Health Care Social Media: Getting Executives on Board (http://goo.gl/rSjmg)

 Published as a whitepaper by the Healthcare Association of New York State, this report describes seven keys to getting hesitant healthcare executives to understand the value of social media. It is designed to help healthcare marketing/communications professionals make the case for implementing a social media strategy within their organizations by addressing business objectives, usage statistics, HIPAA concerns, and reputation management.

Pennsylvania Academy of Family Physicians: PAFP Big 3: Primary Care & Social Media and PAFP Big 3: Primary Care & Advanced Social Media (http://goo.gl/cxQe3)

 The *PAFP BIG 3: Primary Care & Social Media* series focuses on the three biggest social media tools (Facebook, LinkedIn, and Twitter). It provides guidelines for both novices and more experienced users to maximize their online presence through these sites.

PAFP Big 3: Primary Care & Advanced Social Media guides professionals on leveraging their digital footprint. This guide covers some advanced features of Facebook, LinkedIn, and Twitter and introduces YouTube, Skype, and WordPress.

PricewaterhouseCoopers: Social Media "Likes" Healthcare: From Marketing to Social Business (http://goo.gl/P9bYd)

 PricewaterhouseCoopers (PwC) Health Research Institute published a detailed report of social media's impact on the entire healthcare industry. Data were gathered from more than 30 interviews with executives and thought leaders from the biotech industry, pharmaceutical companies, insurers, healthcare provider organizations, patient advocacy organizations, and community health companies. PwC also tracked the social media activity of health organizations and surveyed more than 1000 adults in the United States to look at how they think about and use social media. The report provides insights into new and emerging relationships between consumers and the healthcare industry.

SOCIAL MEDIA BEST PRACTICE RESOURCES

American Congress of Obstetricians and Gynecologists: Social Media Guide (http://goo.gl/zvm5u)

 This 14-page report from American Congress of Obstetricians and Gynecologists provides a helpful overview of how social media can enhance the practice of obstetrics and gynecology. It includes guidelines on blogging and using Facebook and Twitter, as well as social media do's and don'ts, tips to get the best out of social media in the practice, and the use of apps in obstetrics and gynecology.

Bryan Vartabedian, MD, and Joey Spinner, MD: Digital Smarts: A Common Sense Primer for Interns (http://goo.gl/R366T)

 This YouTube presentation was incorporated into the digital professional orientation at Texas Children's Hospital's residency program. Pediatric gastroenterologist Bryan Vartabedian, MD, and second-year resident Joey Spinner, MD, created this practical overview of pearls and pitfalls of social media use.

CDC: Gateway to Health Communication & Social Marketing Practice (http://goo.gl/UuHcP)

 The Centers for Disease Control and Prevention's Gateway to Health Communication & Social Marketing Practice has numerous online resources to help build health communication and social marketing campaigns and programs. It provides tips for analyzing and segmenting an audience, choosing appropriate channels and tools, and evaluating the success of messages and campaigns.

Federation of State Medical Boards: Model Policy Guidelines for the Appropriate Use of Social Media and Social Networking in Medical Practice (http://goo.gl/GRsgS)

 This 17-page guide is the work of a Special Committee on Ethics and Professionalism of the Federation of State Medical Boards (FSMB). It provides "ethical and professional guidance to the FSMB membership with regard to the use of electronic and digital media . . . that may be used to facilitate patient care and nonprofessional interactions." The guidelines cover professional and ethical standards and appropriate use of social media and social networking in medical practice, and provide key definitions and a glossary along with references for further reading.

Ohio State Medical Association: Social Networking and the Medical Practice (http://goo.gl/kb58P)

 The Ohio State Medical Association offers a 10-page social media toolkit to help physicians navigate through the world of online communication. It provides examples of how best to handle certain situations that a physician might encounter when using social media, including whether or not to "friend" a patient. In addition to guidelines for physicians, the toolkit has best practices for social media use in the medical office environment and sample workplace policies.

University of Michigan Health System: Social Media Policy & Toolkit (http://goo.gl/U3OrJ)

 The University of Michigan's social media toolkit provides specific policies for university health system faculty and staff, as well as guidelines for success, consideration for personal use of social media, understanding the risks for healthcare professionals, best practices, and related resources.

Vanderbilt University Medical Center: Social Media Policy and Toolkit (http://goo.gl/zBM2r)

 Vanderbilt University Medical Center (VUMC) was one of the first medical centers in the country to develop a social media policy to guide use of social media by its faculty, staff, and students. While this toolkit is designed to provide social computing guidelines for VUMC faculty, staff, and students engaging in online discourse, it contains guidance on popular platforms, best practices, and participation guidelines that can apply to anyone using social media in medicine.

SAMPLE SOCIAL MEDIA POLICIES

Cleveland Clinic: Social Media Policy (http://goo.gl/T7YZR)

 This page provides a comprehensive social media policy governing the use and posting on any Cleveland Clinic social media site.

KevinMD.com: Terms of Use Agreement (http://goo.gl/cIzpJ)

 This page provides the Terms of Use Agreement created by medical blogger Kevin Pho, MD.

Massachusetts Medical Society: Social Media Guidelines for Physicians (http://goo.gl/M7sib)

 From the viewpoint that social media is professionally appropriate and that it can be an effective way to connect with colleagues, advance professional expertise, educate patients, and enhance the public profile and reputation of the profession, the Massachusetts Medical Society has created guidelines for physicians. The 12-page report covers standards of patient privacy and confidentiality, boundaries of the patient-physician relationship online, professional boundaries, and responsibility for maintaining the profession's code of ethics in online communities.

MD Anderson Cancer Center: Blog Policies and Guidelines (http://goo.gl/5K6wn)

 The MD Anderson Cancerwise blog is an online resource for cancer patients, caregivers, students, and professionals created to offer current expert commentary from bloggers within the institution on treatment, prevention, research, and other pertinent topics. The blog also allows readers to comment and provides an opportunity for staff at MD Anderson to listen to and connect directly with the public. This site details the Terms of Use and provides guidelines for commenting.

University of Maryland Medical Center: Comments Policy and Blog Participation Terms and Conditions (http://goo.gl/aappK)

 This site provides the University of Maryland Medical Center's (UMMC's) official policies for users providing comments on any UMMC social media site.

REPUTATION MANAGEMENT COMPANIES

Reputation.com
www.reputation.com

RepMD
www.repmd.com

eMerit
www.emerit.biz

Healthcare Marketing Center
www.healthcaremarketingcoe.com

Index